Nerve-Related Injuries and Treatments for the Lower Extremity

Editor

STEPHEN L. BARRETT

CLINICS IN PODIATRIC MEDICINE AND SURGERY

www.podiatric.theclinics.com

Consulting Editor
THOMAS ZGONIS

April 2016 • Volume 33 • Number 2

ELSEVIER

1600 John F. Kennedy Boulevard ● Suite 1800 ● Philadelphia, Pennsylvania, 19103-2899

http://www.theclinics.com

CLINICS IN PODIATRIC MEDICINE AND SURGERY Volume 33, Number 2
April 2016 ISSN 0891-8422, ISBN-13: 978-0-323-41769-3

Editor: Jennifer Flynn-Briggs
Developmental Editor: Alison Swety

Clinics in Podiatric Medicine and Surgery (ISSN 0891-8422) is published quarterly by Elsevier Inc., 360 Park Avenue South, New York, NY 10010-1710. Months of issue are January, April, July, and October. Business and Editorial Offices: 1600 John F. Kennedy Blvd., Ste. 1800, Philadelphia, PA 19103-2899. Customer Service Office: 3251 Riverport Lane, Maryland Heights, MO 63043. Periodicals postage paid at New York, NY and additional mailing offices. Subscription prices are $285.00 per year for US individuals, $498.00 per year for US institutions, $100.00 per year for US students and residents, $370.00 per year for Canadian individuals, $602.00 for Canadian institutions, $435.00 for international individuals, $602.00 per year for international institutions and $220.00 per year for Canadian and foreign students/residents. To receive student/resident rate, orders must be accompanied by name of affiliated institution, date of term, and the *signature* of program/residency coordinator on institution letterhead. Orders will be billed at individual rate until proof of status is received. Foreign air speed delivery is included in all *Clinics* subscription prices. All prices are subject to change without notice. POSTMASTER: Send address changes to *Clinics in Podiatric Medicine and Surgery*, Elsevier Health Sciences Division, Subscription Customer Service, 3251 Riverport Lane, Maryland Heights, MO 63043. **Customer Service: 1-800-654-2452 (US). From outside of the US, call 314-447-8871. Fax: 314-447-8029. E-mail: JournalsCustomerService-usa@elsevier.com (for print support); JournalsOnlineSupport-usa@elsevier.com (for online support).**

Reprints. For copies of 100 or more of articles in this publication, please contact the Commercial Reprints Department, Elsevier Inc., 360 Park Avenue South, New York, NY 10010-1710. Tel.: 212-633-3874; Fax: 212-633-3820; E-mail: reprints@elsevier.com.

Clinics in Podiatric Medicine and Surgery is covered in *MEDLINE/PubMed (Index Medicus) and EMBASE/Excerpta Medica*.

CLINICS IN PODIATRIC MEDICINE AND SURGERY

CONSULTING EDITOR
THOMAS ZGONIS, DPM, FACFAS

Contributors

CONSULTING EDITOR

THOMAS ZGONIS, DPM, FACFAS
Professor and Director, Externship and Reconstructive Foot and Ankle Fellowship Programs, Division of Podiatric Medicine and Surgery, Department of Orthopedics, University of Texas Health Science Center San Antonio, San Antonio, Texas

EDITOR

STEPHEN L. BARRETT, DPM, MBA, FAENS, FACFAS
Adjunct Professor, Arizona School of Podiatric Medicine, Midwestern University College of Health Sciences, Glendale, Arizona; CEO, Innovative Neuropathy Treatment Institute, Phoenix, Arizona

AUTHORS

JAMES C. ANDERSON, DPM, FAENS, FACFAS, FASPS
Anderson Podiatry Center for Nerve Pain, Fort Collins, Colorado

STEPHEN L. BARRETT, DPM, MBA, FAENS, FACFAS
Adjunct Professor, Arizona School of Podiatric Medicine, Midwestern University College of Health Sciences, Glendale, Arizona; CEO, Innovative Neuropathy Treatment Institute, Phoenix, Arizona

RICHARD T. BRAVER, DPM, FACFAS, FASPS, FAAPSM
Attending, Department of Podiatry, Hackensack University Medical Center, Hackensack, New Jersey; Team Podiatric Physician Consultant, Montclair State University, Montclair, New Jersey; Fairleigh Dickinson University, Teaneck, New Jersey; William Paterson University, Wayne, New Jersey; Scientific Advisory Board Member, Runner's World Magazine, Emmaus, Pennsylvania

PETER J. BREGMAN, DPM, FAENS, FACFAS
Board Certified by The American Board of Foot and Ankle Surgery, Bregman Peripheral Neuropathy Center of Las Vegas, Foot, Ankle, and Hand Center of Las Vegas, Las Vegas, Nevada

A. LEE DELLON, MD, PhD
Professor of Plastic Surgery and Neurosurgery, Johns Hopkins University, Baltimore, Maryland

ORLANDO MERCED-O'NEIL, BS, RN, CTBS
Associate Director of Medical Services; Microsurgery Instructor, AxoGen, Inc, Alachua, Florida

DAVID SCOTT NICKERSON, MD, FAAOS
Consultant, NE Wyoming Wound Clinic, Sheridan Memorial Hospital, Sheridan, Wyoming

ROBERT G. PARKER, DPM, FACFAS, FAENS, FASPS
Immediate Past President and Fellow Association of Extremity Nerve Surgeons;
Co-Founder, Harris County Podiatric Resident Program; Fellow, American College of Foot
and Ankle Surgeons; Diplomate, Past Examiner, American Board of Foot and Ankle
Surgery, Houston, Texas

MARK SCHUENKE, PhD
Associate Professor of Anatomy, University of New England College of Osteopathic
Medicine, Biddeford, Maine

JAMES P. WILTON, DPM, FAENS, FACFAS
Department of Orthopedics, New England Peripheral Nerve Center, Valley Regional
Hospital, Claremont, New Hampshire

DWAYNE S. YAMASAKI, PhD
Medtronic, Jacksonville, Florida

Contents

Burning sensation in the feet is a common problem encountered in podiatric medicine. When this pain is bilateral, symmetric, and includes the top and bottom of both feet, small nerve fiber involvement must be considered in the differential diagnosis. With the now available, in-office, skin biopsy quantification of intraepidermal nerve fibers, documentation of the presence of small fiber involvement in the pain mechanism is possible. Technical details of performing the skin biopsy are reviewed and the legal implications of a positive abnormal skin biopsy for intraepidermal nerve fibers is discussed.

A focused lower extremity neurologic evaluation aids in the diagnosis of lower extremity nerve pathology. Injuries to the peripheral neural infrastructure can result in chronic neuropathic pain and discomfort. The most common etiologies of chronic neuropathic pain are from peripheral distal pathologies. A complete lower extremity neurologic evaluation includes sensory, motor, and deep tendon reflexes. Additional specific attention to the geographic anatomic testing of peripheral sensory and motor nerves is essential in eliciting a correct etiologic diagnosis for peripheral neural pain and dysfunction.

There is a large reservoir of leprosy patients, no longer contagious, due to multidrug therapy, who are considered cured and are becoming increasingly disabled due to progressive chronic nerve entrapment in the upper and lower extremities. After a review of the history of understanding leprous neuropathy, an approach is outlined based on the approach taken to relieve pain and restore sensation that prevents ulcers and amputations in diabetics with neuropathy and superimposed nerve compressions. The results of the first application of this approach in an indigenous area for leprosy, Guayaquil, Ecuador, is discussed with implications for international care of this neglected patient population.

> Increased tissue pressure within a fascial compartment may be the result
> from any increase in volume within its contents, or any decrease in size of
> the fascial covering or its distensibility. This may lead to symptoms of leg
> tightness, pain, or numbness brought about by exercise. There are multi-
> ple differential diagnoses of exercise induced leg pain. The proper diagno-
> ses of chronic exertional compartment syndrome (CECS) is made by a
> careful history and by exclusion of other maladies and confirmed by
> compartment syndrome testing, as detailed in this text. Surgical fascito-
> mies for the anterior, lateral, superficial, and deep posterior compartments
> are described in detail along with ancillary procedures for chronic shin
> splints that should allow the athlete to return to competitive activity.

> Painful recurrent stump neuroma presents a common clinical problem
> following the transection of a nerve after initial interdigital neuroma exci-
> sion, but there is no gold standard of treatment. A patient presented with
> pain symptoms consistent with recurrent intermetatarsal stump neuroma
> after undergoing previous surgery to excise a Hauser neuroma. The recur-
> rent stump neuroma was excised and the resulting nerve was capped and
> implantation into intrinsic muscle. Postoperatively, the patient experienced
> a complete resolution of pain and return of normal function. This article dis-
> cusses capping material characteristics and considers the factors that
> may contribute to clinical success.

 Video content accompanies this article at http://www.podiatric.
theclinics.com

> The superficial peroneal nerve is now known as the superficial fibular nerve
> (SFN). Identification and treatment of entrapment of the SFN are important
> topics of discussion for foot and ankle surgeons, because overlooking the
> diagnosis can lead to permanent nerve damage. With the proper tools and
> skills, surgeons are able to help patients with symptomatic SFN entrap-
> ment, patients who often present in some degree of desperation, with
> the peripheral nerve surgeon as a last resort.

 Video content accompanies this article at http://www.podiatric.
theclinics.com

> This article describes the benefits of intraoperative neurophysiologic
> monitoring (IONM) and proposes methods for integration into nerve

decompression procedures. Standard procedures for intraoperative nerve monitoring (IONM) are illustrated as they would apply to the 3 nerve tunnels that have significant motor components within the lower extremity.

Nerve decompression is effective and safe for dealing with the pain and numbness symptoms of the frequent nerve compression entrapments in diabetic symmetric peripheral neuropathy (DSPN). Evidence has accumulated of balance and stability improvements and protection against diabetic foot ulceration, recurrence, and its complication cascade. Nerve decompression proffers significant benefit versus the large socioeconomic costs of DSPN complications. Advancing understanding of the mechanism of nerve compression and altered axonal activity in diabetes clarifies the basis of clinical benefit. Clinicians should seek out and recognize nerve entrapments and consider advising nerve decompression for relief of DSPN symptoms and prevention of complications.

This article thoroughly describes the clinical examination and treatment of common fibular (peroneal) nerve compression. Aspects discussed include the anatomy of the nerve, cause of entrapment, symptoms associated with impairment, and a surgical approach to decompress the entrapped nerve. The standard protocol for decompression as it would apply to the common fibular nerve tunnel is illustrated.

This case illustrates the complexity and interrelationship of osseous pathology with peripheral nerve entrapment and neuromata. The patient had an iatrogenic nerve injury of a branch of the medial dorsal cutaneous nerve causing her painful scar. Secondarily, she developed an injury to her common peroneal nerve from the cast immobilization, resulting in palsy/drop foot. The tarsal tunnel entrapment was likely a sequela of the cast immobilization and chronic swelling. Her postoperative chronic pain was compounded by the failure to use grommets with the polymeric silicon (Silastic) implant at the initial surgery, leading to a breakdown of the implant with subsequent detritic synovitis.

CLINICS IN PODIATRIC MEDICINE AND SURGERY

RELATED INTEREST

Orthopedic Clinics, April 2016 (Vol. 47, Issue 2)
Common Complications in Orthopedics
James H. Calandruccio, Benjamin J. Grear, Benjamin M. Mauck, Jeffrey R. Sawyer, Patrick C. Toy, and John C. Weinlein, *Editors*
Available at: http://www.orthopedic.theclinics.com/

THE CLINICS ARE AVAILABLE ONLINE!
Access your subscription at:
www.theclinics.com

Foreword

Nerve-Related Injuries and Treatments for the Lower Extremity

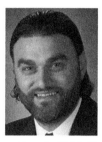

Thomas Zgonis, DPM, FACFAS
Consulting Editor

This issue of *Clinics in Podiatric Medicine and Surgery* is focused on nerve-related injuries, entrapments, and treatments of the lower extremity. From small-fiber neuropathy and skin biopsy techniques to chronic nerve compression in the diabetic patient, this issue covers a wide range of neurologic conditions for the reconstructive surgeon. Great emphasis is given to the detailed lower extremity neurologic examination and surgical nerve decompression for diabetic neuropathic foot conditions.

In addition, intraoperative nerve monitoring as a surgical tool during surgical nerve decompression and an overview of chronic exertional compartment syndrome treated with fasciotomies in the athlete are well covered by our invited authors. Finally, I would like to thank the Guest Editor, Dr Stephen L. Barrett, invited authors, editorial board members, and readers for their continuous support of and dedication to *Clinics in Podiatric Medicine and Surgery*.

Thomas Zgonis, DPM, FACFAS
Externship and Reconstructive Foot and Ankle Fellowship Programs
Division of Podiatric Medicine and Surgery
Department of Orthopedics
University of Texas Health Science Center San Antonio
7703 Floyd Curl Drive-MSC 7706
San Antonio, TX 78229, USA

E-mail address:
zgonis@uthscsa.edu

Clin Podiatr Med Surg 33 (2016) xi
http://dx.doi.org/10.1016/j.cpm.2016.01.002
0891-8422/16/$ – see front matter © 2016 Published by Elsevier Inc.

podiatric.theclinics.com

Preface

Peripheral Nerve Surgery— A New Subspecialty

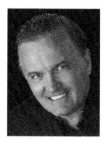

Stephen L. Barrett, DPM, MBA, FAENS, FACFAS
Editor

As a subspecialty, Podiatric Surgery has emerged to encompass an almost incomprehensible level of knowledge and now has many subspecialties within the subspecialty– for example, wound care, limb salvage, Charcot reconstruction, and biomechanics, just to name a few. Sadly, there has been a very important, but largely unrecognized subspecialty that has existed for more than a decade and a half, and that is of lower extremity peripheral nerve surgery. This "new" subspecialty is growing quickly and is gaining significant recognition not only by our profession but also by neurology, endocrinology, family practitioners, and pain management specialists. This high level of knowledge, expertise, and the vast breadth of this body of work have been increasingly recognized since the formation of the Association of Extremity Nerve Surgeons, which is an affiliate organization of the American Podiatric Medical Association. It is composed of MDs, DOs, and DPMs working in concert to improve patient outcomes with lower extremity pain and pathology. As the immediate past president of this association, it is my honor to bring this issue dedicated to peripheral nerve pathology and surgery to the podiatric profession.

Stephen L. Barrett, DPM, MBA, FAENS, FACFAS
Innovative Neuropathy Treatment Institute
16601 North 40th Street
Suite 110
Phoenix, AZ 85032, USA

E-mail address:
slbarrettpod@me.com

Clin Podiatr Med Surg 33 (2016) xiii
http://dx.doi.org/10.1016/j.cpm.2016.01.001
0891-8422/16/$ – see front matter © 2016 Published by Elsevier Inc.

Small Fiber Neuropathy
Differential Diagnosis and Treatment Implications

Stephen L. Barrett, DPM, MBA[a], A. Lee Dellon, MD, PhD[b],*

KEYWORDS

- Small fiber neuropathy • Intraepidermal nerve ending • Skin biopsy

KEY POINTS

- When the unmyelinated and small myelinated nerve fibers are symptomatic, patients' complaints are of burning extremity pain.
- Skin biopsy is now standardized to identify abnormal intraepidermal nerve fiber density, which correlates with a patient's small fiber disease.
- *Pure small fiber neuropathy is rare.* Treatment with neuropathic drugs and topical creams is appropriate. Nerve decompression is not appropriate.
- Abnormal cutaneous pressure or vibratory thresholds and/or abnormal nerve conduction velocity or distal latency document that pure small fiber neuropathy is *not* present, because these are tests of large fiber function.
- Chronic nerve compression and mixed (large and small) fiber neuropathy, as in diabetes, also can give an abnormal skin biopsy for intraepidermal nerve fibers, in which case, nerve decompression surgery may be appropriate.

INTRODUCTION

Burning sensation in the feet is a common problem encountered in podiatric medicine. When this pain is bilateral, symmetric, and includes the top and bottom of both feet, small nerve fiber involvement must be considered in the differential diagnosis. These "small nerve fibers" include the unmyelinated C-fibers and the thinly myelinated group A-delta fibers, which transmit perception of hot and cold and burning or itching pain.[1] *Small nerve fibers do not transmit the perception of numbness.* It is the large, myelinated A-beta fibers that transmit the perception of touch, including vibratory perception and pressure perception.[1] Abnormal perception of touch is described as numbness, not pain. Numbness can be described as unpleasant, or paresthesias, but is not burning pain. Documentation of small fiber function requires quantitative sensory

[a] Arizona School of Podiatric Medicine, Midwestern University College of Health Sciences, Glendale, AZ, USA; [b] Johns Hopkins University, Baltimore, MD, USA
* Corresponding author. 1122 Kenilworth Drive, Suite 18, Towson, MD 21204.
E-mail address: aldellon@dellon.com

Clin Podiatr Med Surg 33 (2016) 185–189
http://dx.doi.org/10.1016/j.cpm.2015.12.001
0891-8422/16/$ – see front matter © 2016 Elsevier Inc. All rights reserved.

testing with cutaneous warmth or cold thresholds, but this testing is not usually available.[2] Documentation of large fiber function is commonly done with either the Semmes-Weinstein monofilaments, to give an estimate of a range for 1-point static touch, or with the pressure-specified sensory device, to give a direct measurement of the pressure required to discriminate 1-point from 2-point static touch.[2] Traditional electrodiagnostic testing of the sensory conduction velocity or the distal sensory latency are also traditional measures of large fiber function.[2] A computer-assisted sensory evaluation with the CASE IV, developed by the Neurology Department at the Mayo Clinic, which incorporates thermal testing, vibration testing, and 1-point static testing thresholds has been used to quantitate both small and large fiber function demonstrating them to be abnormal in patients with diabetes and with subclinical problems related to running,[3–5] but this device is not generally available.

The realization that the terminal endings of the small fibers innervate the skin in the epidermis, lead the way to a quantitative measurement of these endings in a skin biopsy. This testing was developed and standardized by the Neurology Department at Johns Hopkins Hospital and published in 1998.[6] Decreased intraepidermal nerve fiber density correlated with the presence of pain in this study. The presence of pure small fiber neuropathy is rare, with this same neurology group reporting on just 32 such patients in their now classic article on this disease.[7]

Prevalence and incidence of pure small fiber neuropathy has been reported recently in the Netherlands: it was found in 55 patients over a 5-year time period in a clinic devoted to the treatment of these types of problems, with an incidence of 11.7 per 100,000 population.[8]

An abnormal intraepidermal nerve fiber density report from a skin biopsy must be considered as a finding, not as a diagnosis of pure small fiber neuropathy. Chronic nerve compression and the commonest forms of polyneuropathy also can have decreased intraepidermal nerve fiber density.

DIFFERENTIAL DIAGNOSIS

Does the presence of abnormal intraepidermal nerve fibers exclude the diagnosis of mixed fiber neuropathy, or of chronic nerve compression, or of neuropathy with superimposed chronic nerve compression? It is clear from the following articles, including the original article from the Johns Hopkins Neurology group, that many forms of neuropathy have both large and small fiber abnormalities.[6,7,9,10] It is also clear from studies on humans with chronic nerve compression,[11–13] and on rats with chronic nerve compression,[14] that small fibers are affected in these conditions too: chronic nerve compression has abnormalities of both large and small nerve fibers.

A positive skin biopsy for decreased intraepidermal nerve fibers is, therefore, consistent with the diagnosis of pure small fiber neuropathy, mixed fiber neuropathy, or chronic nerve compression. A differential diagnosis should be included in the skin biopsy reporting format, and understood by the physician ordering that test.[15]

TECHNIQUE FOR A SKIN BIOPSY TO EVALUATE SMALL FIBER DENSITY

What you will need:
- Betadine
- Small pair of dissecting scissors
- Disposable forceps
- 3-mm punch biopsy
- Labeled vial
- 5.0 nylon suture (optional) (**Fig. 1A**)

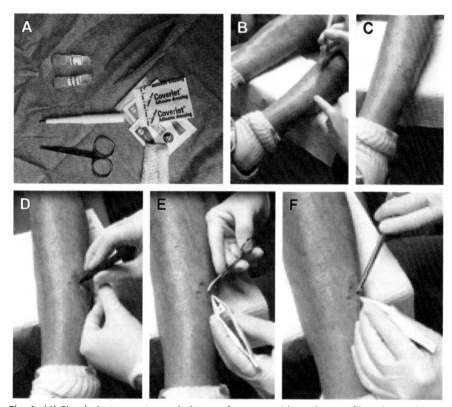

Fig. 1. (A) Simple instruments needed to perform an epidermal nerve fiber density biopsy including a small 3-mm punch biopsy and disposable forceps. (B) For a calf biopsy the usual anatomical site is about 10-cm proximal from the lateral malleolus. (C) The area is prepped with povidone-iodine, after a small local anesthetic wheal is raised. (D) By twisting the punch biopsy all the way through the dermis a good specimen can be obtained. (E) Careful attention must be made not to "squeeze" the specimen. The forceps should be used in a closed fashion as seen here to lift the specimen from the subcutaneous fat. Any attachment to the subcutaneous fat needs to be cut to remove the specimen cleanly. (F) We recommend placing a 5-0 nylon suture to close the biopsy site.

Step 1: Apply block of lidocaine with epinephrine 10–12 cm proximal to the lateral malleolus. Infiltrate slowly. You should raise up a nice wheal in the area (**Fig. 1**B).

Step 2: Swab area with Betadine (**Fig. 1**C).

Step 3: Take a 3-mm punch, using a slight side-to-side rolling/twisting motion into skin.

Technique Tip: The optimal sample will be symmetrical in shape. To achieve this, insert the punch until you are into the subcutaneous space (you will feel a slight give as the tissue density changes). Slowly roll the punch from side to side several times to loosen the tissue for removal (**Fig. 1**D).

Step 4: Use dissection scissors and forceps to remove the sample, being careful not to squeeze the epidermal sample. Place in vial of Zamboni fluid.

Technique Tip: When removing the sample, you want to be sure to keep some of the subcutaneous fat intact. Also, DO NOT squeeze the sample. Use the forceps like a lever underneath the sample, rather than grasping the sample itself. This ensures the epidermal nerve fibers are not crushed (**Fig. 1**E).

Step 5: Turn vial to ensure specimen is well covered by preservative.

Step 6: For optimal outcomes, it is recommended to put in a 5.0 nylon stitch (**Fig. 1F**).

Step 7: Cover with bandage.

Step 8: Give patient written instructions on taking care of the biopsy site.

Step 9: Send out for staining and read by a dermatopathologist.

Note: Performing a second distal/plantar foot biopsy is recommended, especially when the patient complains of significant plantar numbness in the forefoot. This can give tremendous insight into length dependent axonal neuropathy. The procedure is the same, except the location is the plantar aspect of the foot in a non–weight-bearing area proximal to the first and second metatarsal heads.

TREATMENT CONSIDERATIONS

The patient with burning pain in the feet, also often described as stepping on hot coals or electric shocks, or the patient who wishes to put feet into ice water, must be considered to have small fiber dysfunction. This can be documented with temperature thresholds if available, but most likely will have an abnormal skin biopsy demonstrated by decreased intraepidermal nerve fibers in the calf or foot compared with the thigh. If large fiber function is demonstrated to be normal by electrodiagnostic testing or vibratory or pressure thresholds, then treatment with neuropathic medication and topical creams containing a combination of gabapentin, capsaicin, ketamine, and lidocaine is most appropriate. These patients are not surgical candidates for nerve decompression.

The patient with burning pain who *also* has numbness, and who has an abnormal intraepidermal nerve fiber density found on skin biopsy of the calf/foot compared with the ankle, may be a candidate for nerve decompression *IF* there is also a positive Tinel sign over a known anatomic site of narrowing, like the tibial nerve in the tarsal tunnel, or tenderness over the common peroneal nerve at the fibular neck, and *IF* there is also documented large fiber abnormality on either electrodiagnostic testing or cutaneous pressure or vibratory threshold.

In the presence of physical findings consistent with a chronic nerve compression, a positive skin biopsy for abnormal intraepidermal nerve fibers is NOT a contraindication for surgical decompression of the peripheral nerve at this anatomic site.

SUMMARY

It may be concluded then that, in the patient with symptoms of numbness and pain, who has had an abnormal skin biopsy for intraepidermal nerve fibers, that the presence of large fiber dysfunction can be demonstrated by electrodiagnostic testing, or quantitative sensory testing, to prove that the patient does not have pure small fiber neuropathy. If the patient's history fits with a chronic nerve compression, and their physical findings document localized signs of compression at a known site of anatomic narrowing (positive Tinel sign), then surgical decompression is appropriate even in the presence of an abnormal skin biopsy for intraepidermal nerve fibers.

REFERENCES

1. Dellon AL. Evaluation of sensibility and re-education of sensation in the hand. Baltimore (MD): Williams and Wilkins Publication; 1981.
2. Dellon AL. Somatosensory testing and rehabilitation. Bethesda (MD): American Occupational Therapy Association Publication; 1997.

3. Dyck PJ, Karnes J, Bushek W, et al. Computer assisted sensory examination to detect and quantitate sensory deficit in diabetic neuropathy. Neurobehav Toxicol Teratol 1983;5(6):697–704.
4. Dyck PJ, Classen SM, Stevens JC, et al. Assessment of nerve damage in the feet of long-distance runners. Mayo Clin Proc 1987;62(7):568–72.
5. Dyck PJ, Zimmerman IR, Johnson DM, et al. A standard test of heat-pain responses using CASE IV. J Neurol Sci 1996;136(1–2):54–63.
6. McArthur JC, Stocks EA, Hauer P, et al. Epidermal nerve fiber density: normative reference range and diagnostic efficiency. Arch Neurol 1998;55:1513–20.
7. Holland NR, Crawford TO, Bauer P, et al. Small-fiber sensory neuropathies: clinical course and neuropatholgy of idiopathic cases. Ann Neurol 1998;44: 47–59.
8. Peters MJ, Bakkers M, Kerkies IS, et al. Incidence and prevalence of small-fiber neuropathy; a survey in the Netherlands. Neurology 2013;81:1356–60.
9. Hermann DH, Griffin JW, Hauer P, et al. Epidural nerve fiber density and sural nerve morphometry in peripheral neuropathies. Neurology 1999;53:1634–40.
10. Saperstein DS, Levine TD, Levin M, et al. Usefulness of skin biopsies in the evaluation and management of patients with suspected small fiber neuropathies. Int J Neurosci 2013;123:38–41.
11. Mackinnon SE, Dellon AL, Hudson AR, et al. Chronic human nerve compression: a histological assessment. Neuropathol Appl Neurobiol 1986;12:547–65.
12. Mackinnon SE, Dellon AL, Hudson AR, et al. Histopathology of compression of the superficial radial nerve in the forearm. J Hand Surg 1986;11A:206–10.
13. Schmidt AB. The relationship of nerve fiber pathology to sensory function in entrapment neuropathy. Brain 2014;1–14. http://dx.doi.org/10.1093/brain/awu288.
14. Schmid AB, Coppieters MS, Ruitenberg MJ. Local and remote immune-mediated inflammation after mild peripheral nerve compression in rats. J Neuropathol Exp Neurol 2013;72:662–80.
15. Dellon AL. Abnormal skin biopsy for intra-epidermal nerve fibers; when decreased "small nerve fibers" is not "small fiber neuropathy". Microsurgery 2015;35. http://dx.doi.org/10.1002/micr.22372.

Lower Extremity Focused Neurologic Examination

James P. Wilton, DPM

KEYWORDS

- Nerve • Sensory • Motor • Injury • Dysesthesia • Pain

KEY POINTS

- A focused lower extremity neurologic examination is based on motor examination, sensory examination and deep tendon reflexes. The physician should review all prior examinations and test results for a complete medical evaluation.
- It is common in clinical practice to encounter patients presenting with chronic limb pain.
- A thorough and complete lower extremity neurologic examination will aid in the development of a differential diagnosis of neuropathic pain and limb dysfunction.
- The end result will aid in the differential diagnosis of neuropathic pain and limb dysfunction.
- The practitioner should be able to differentiate between lower extremity peripheral nerve injury, peripheral neuropathy, lumbosacral nerve pathology, upper motor neuron disease, and central nervous system pathology.

Medical training today has become so compartmentalized between the medical specialties that a patient presenting with limb pain or dysfunction may have several different diagnostic labels attributed to the etiology of their problem. When a practitioner who primarily works with the structural limb components associated with long bones, muscles, tendons, ligaments, and joints evaluates a patient with limb pain, he approaches the patient with different diagnostic eyes than the practitioner who primarily works with the medical causes of pain. A podiatric foot and ankle surgeon, orthopedic foot and ankle surgeon, general orthopedist, vascular surgeon, plastic surgeon, physiatrist, pain specialist, family practitioner, pediatrician, internist, and neurologist all bring different skill sets to the diagnostic process of peripheral limb pain. Although the first 2 years of medical training for all of these medical practitioners are essentially indistinguishable from a basic science standpoint and physical examination skill set standpoint, the following 2 years of medical school and subsequent residency and fellowship training are so highly compartmentalized and specialized

Department of Orthopedics, New England Peripheral Nerve Center, Valley Regional Hospital, 241 Elm Street, Claremont, NH 03743, USA
E-mail address: James.Wilton@VRH.org

Clin Podiatr Med Surg 33 (2016) 191–202
http://dx.doi.org/10.1016/j.cpm.2015.12.008   **podiatric.theclinics.com**
0891-8422/16/$ – see front matter © 2016 Elsevier Inc. All rights reserved.

that commonalities in diagnostic approaches are very varied. Midlevel providers such as physician assistants and nurse practitioners also have very diverse clinical training and bring different education and experience to the arena of clinical examination.

The Association of Extremity Nerve Surgeons devotes this article to the "hands-on" peripheral neurologic examination developed for the students in the basic and advanced peripheral nerve surgery courses. It is not the purview of this paper to delve into the lower extremity orthopedic, dermatologic or vascular examination because the assumption will be made that most practitioners reading this monograph have adequate skill sets in these components of the clinical assessment. The greatest weakness that we faculty have observed in the board-certified surgeons who partic-ipate in these specialized peripheral nerve surgical training courses is not the individ-ual surgical skills needed to perform peripheral nerve surgery, but the lack of a competent and complete initial diagnostic "hands-on" neurologic workup of patient's experiencing chronic pain (Robert Parker, DPM FAENS FACFAS, Houston, Texas, personal communication, May 2015).

These gifted lower extremity surgeons who can technically perform complex recon-structive foot and ankle surgery have, to some degree, lost some of the basic skills that they learned as first and second year medical students in the clinical examination of a patient. Through the development of highly specialized skill sets in their residency and fellowship training, they have relegated many components of the basic peripheral neurologic examination to antiquity. Nonsurgical specialists that take these training courses also benefit from learning these clinical neurologic examinations because they will refine and develop new skill sets to help them diagnosis complex patients experiencing chronic limb pain that present to their practices.

The clinical examination must focus on past medical, past surgical, and past trau-matic history in addition to the hands-on testing of the peripheral nervous system. In most cases, patients who present to podiatric foot and ankle surgeons for evalua-tion and treatment of chronic limb pain have been worked up thoroughly through mul-tiple layers of medical care. It is not uncommon to initially evaluate the patient with chronic limb pain who has seen their family practitioner, orthopedic surgeon, physiat-rist, neurologist, and pain physician. Medical records including family and social his-tory, past medical and surgical histories, diagnostic imaging studies, hematologic studies, and electrodiagnostic studies are usually readily available for review. It is very helpful to take the approach to allow your hands-on clinical neurologic examina-tion to be the foundation of your diagnostic decision making process.[1] Although pre-vious diagnostic testing and studies can be helpful, they are only a piece of the diagnostic pie. If the clinical approach is cursory in nature and major components of the neurologic examination are not performed, then conclusions and the final diag-nosis may be based on false or inaccurate data.[2] It is the ultimate goal of a competent and complete lower extremity neurologic evaluation to develop a working diagnosis and to also see if referral to medical practitioners in other fields, diagnostic imaging or additional electrodiagnostic testing is needed.

Unfortunately, the 14th-century principal of *Lex Parsimoniae* or Occam's Razor comes in play far too many times by medical specialists in developing the diagnosis and etiology for chronic peripheral nerve pain. This medieval principal states that, when multiple hypotheses are given for a problem, the simplest solution should be selected. This myopic view concerning complex problems invariably leads to an incor-rect diagnosis (William Ericson FAAOS, MD, Seattle, Washington, personal communi-cation, July 2013).

Complex clinical presentations of chronic limb pain invariably are not of a simple etiologic origin but derive out of complicated scenarios. It is only through a complete and thorough hands-on peripheral neurologic examination that the evaluating physician can have a reasonable chance at arriving at the correct diagnosis, which in turn will lead to an effective treatment plan. Add to the milieu the patient who is involved in a worker's compensation case, civil or criminal legal proceedings, or disability determination case, and the ability of the examining practitioner to develop a correct diagnosis can be of paramount importance and can also be extremely challenging.

CLINICAL EXAMINATION

Initial clinical neurologic examination primarily involves a dialogue with the patient regarding the nature of the presenting problem. A thorough "medical interrogation," keeping the patient focused on the presenting issues, is a difficult clinical skill to master. If left to their own devices, many patients speak at length about their hypotheses concerning both causation and diagnosis of their presenting problems. Keeping the dialogue both on track and point specific with both initial closed ended and then open-ended questions is crucial to an effective examination. It is of utmost importance to elicit from the patient how their specific presenting problems affect the quality of their life and to record this information. Difficulties in performing activities in their social life and in their own occupation are very important to understand because they may present a barrier to effective treatment or unrealistic expectations of final treatment outcomes by the patient.

Observing and inspecting the patient for their outward general appearance and also functional status of the limbs can be performed watching the patient entering and exiting the treatment room.[3] It is also helpful if possible to personally observe or have a staff member observe the patient leave the office and see if there are gait pattern changes when they are not under direct observation by the physician. It is very interesting to observe hand gestures of the patient describing the geographic area of their pain. Clinical experience has shown that patients who localize their hand gestures to a small geographic area indicating their pain location seem to do much better in evaluation and subsequent treatment than those patients who demonstrate their pain location with hand gestures as a global area from the toes to the waist (Ivan Ducic MD PhD, Mclean, Virginia, personal communication, May 2011).

In this part of the examination, one can also evaluate muscle tone, spasticity, and atrophy in the thighs, legs, and intrinsic muscles of the feet, as well as any abnormalities in gait pattern such as a steppage or a drop foot type gait. Can tremors or fasciculations within the larger muscle groups be observed? Does the geographic area of pain correspond with 1 discrete structure or are multiple areas affected either ipsilaterally or contralaterally?

Knowledge of the variability of peripheral neural pathways is of utmost importance in understanding pain transmission. The differentiation of sensory anatomic innervation patterns as one moves distally from the spinal cord to the periphery of the limb can vary greatly and can complicate identification of specific pain generators.[4,5]

MOTOR EXAMINATION

The motor examination is involved primarily with strength testing of the muscles surrounding the hips, thighs, legs, and intrinsic muscles of the feet. It is not uncommon for medical reports to indicate that certain groups of muscles function at normal levels when tested as a group and subsequent evaluation of individual muscles in the group showed different gradations of weakness. It is because of this that we recommend testing individual muscles in muscle groups to get a clear and concise picture of muscle innervation patterns.[6] Subtle differences in motor strength among muscles in 1 muscle group may be a clinical indication of a specific neural problem.

For example, in common fibular nerve entrapment syndromes at the fibular canal in the proximal lateral leg, it is commonly noted that the extensor hallucis longus muscle may have a 1 or 2 grade muscle weakness and the other extensor muscles innervated in the anterior group such as the tibialis anterior, extensor digitorum longus, and peroneus brevis and longus muscles may have a normal 5 over 5 muscle grade. Anatomically the common fibular nerve distally passes through the fibular canal and divides into the deep fibular and superficial fibular nerves. The motor branch to the extensor hallucis longus muscle originating off of the deep fibular nerve passes over a sharp anterior border on the fibula and is easily compressed against the bony surface. Although the patient may have a 5 over 5 dorsiflexion test at the ankle in globalized muscle group testing, significant motor weaknesses can be observed in the extensor hallucis longus muscle when tested independently. The tibialis anterior and peroneal brevis and longus muscles are generally affected after the extensor hallucis longus and extensor digitorum longus muscles in a nontraumatic compression/entrapment syndrome.

Many testing and grading systems for muscles are used clinically and we teach the manual muscle testing grading system based on 0 through 5. In ranges 2 through 5, the clinician can add a plus or minus to further describe weaknesses or strength within those individual muscle grades:

0 denotes no visible or palpable muscle contraction;
1 denotes visible or palpable contraction with no motion;
2 denotes full range of motion gravity eliminated;
3 denotes full range of motion against gravity;
4 denotes full range of motion against gravity, moderate resistance; and
5 denotes full range of motion against gravity, maximal resistance.

Lower extremity muscle testing can easily be performed on an orthopedic table. Initial visual examination should note muscle tone, symmetry of muscles between the extremities, bulk, atrophy, tremors, or fasciculations. A gait examination can also be included at the end of the session. Manual testing starts at the hip and ends with the foot with the muscles delineated in **Figs. 1** and **2A–I** being examined against resistance.

DEEP TENDON REFLEXES

The reflex arc is a combination of sensory and motor signals produced after a defined stimulus. The reflex is composed of the contraction of a muscle in response to a quick stretching of a tendon by means of a percussion hammer. Spindle cells in the tendon are stretched initially by the percussion stimulus and this causes the afferent neuron to fire in a proximal direction, thus stimulating proximal alpha motor neurons in the anterior horn of the spinal cord. This efferent neuron now causes the distal contraction of the muscle that is, being stimulated. To obtain a valid deep tendon reflex, the patient should be relaxed and comfortable. The preferred patient position is sitting on the orthopedic table with the legs hanging off of the side. To elicit a good response, it may necessitate the patient pulling their hands together to distract himself or herself or repositioning the limb being examined to prevent tension on the muscle being tested. If the patient is tense, deep tendon reflexes may not be attainable. Abnormalities in reflex action can give insights into integrity and function of the peripheral nervous system at many levels.

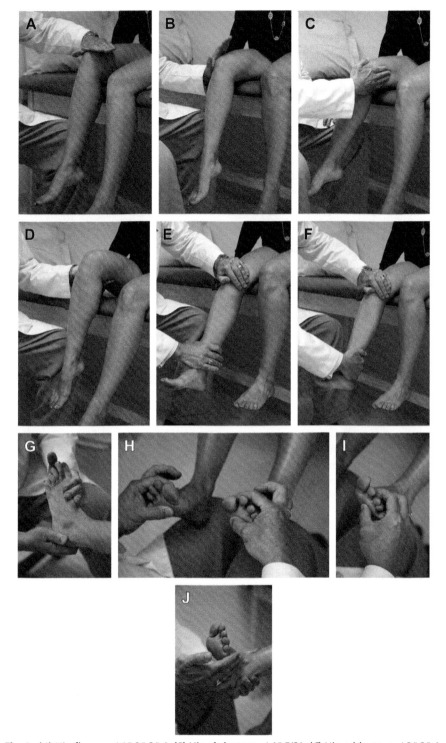

Fig. 1. (*A*) Hip flexors—L1/L2/L3/L4. (*B*) Hip abductors—L4/L5/S1. (*C*) Hip adductors—L2/L3/L4. (*D*) Hip extensors—L2/L3/L4. (*E*) Quadriceps—L2/L3/L4. (*F*) Hamstrings—L4/L5/S1. (*G*) Tibialis anterior—L4/L5. (*H*) Extensor hallucis longus—L5/S1. (*I*) Extensor digitorum longus—L5/S1. (*J*) Peroneus brevis—L5/S1.

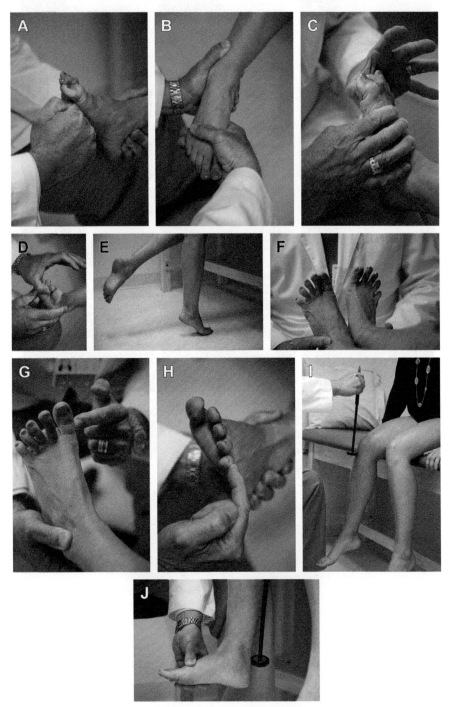

Fig. 2. (*A*). Peroneus longus—L5/S1. (*B*) Tibialis posterior—L4/L5. (*C*) Flexor hallucis longus—L5/S1/S2. (*D*) Flexor digitorum longus—L5/S1/S2. (*E*) Gastrocnemius/soleus—S1/S2. (*F*) Intrinsic muscles of the foot—L5/S1/S2. (*G*) Abductor hallucis—L5/S1. (*H*) Abductor digiti minimi—S2/S3. (*I*) Patellar reflex—L2/L3/L4 nerve roots. (*J*) Achilles reflex—S1/S2 nerve roots.

Our preferred reflex hammer is the Queens Square Hammer named after the famous Queens Square National Hospital for Neurology and Neurosurgery in London, England. It gives a reproducible stimulus for deep tendon reflex testing and is manually easy to use in varying patient examination positions. A simple flick of the wrist combined with the timbre of the hammer arm generates the correct mechanical stimulus to elicit a deep tendon reflex (**Figs. 2I, J, and 3A**).

Deep tendon reflexes are graded as follows:

0—Absent response–abnormal;
1+—Hypoactive response; may be normal or abnormal;
2+—Normal response;
3+—Hyperactive/brisk response; may be normal or abnormal;
4+—Hyperactive reflex with clonus, abnormal; and
5+—Sustained clonus, abnormal.

SENSORY EXAMINATION

Components of the sensory examination of the lower extremities are evaluation of light touch appreciation, sharp and dull discrimination, 2-point discrimination, vibratory perception, percussion, and position sense. Light moving touch against the skin with the patient's eyes closed compares similar areas of sensory innervation on contralateral leg and foot surfaces. A scale of 0 of 10 indicating no sensation through 10 of 10 indicating full sensation is used.

Sharp and Dull Discrimination

Dermatomal tracts and individual peripheral nerve pathways can be tested with a Whartenberg wheel comparing contralateral limbs and other independent ipsilateral nerve tracts against each other. We recommend starting with the index finger and having the eyes open so the patient will clearly understand that this is not a painful stimulus. The patient will then close their eyes for light touch and sharp and dull testing on the lower extremities. This information elicited from this testing can be both qualitative and quantitative in nature. The presence or absence of sensation and qualitative differences in sensory appreciation can be significant findings with peripheral nerve injury (**Figs. 3B–J and 4A–C**).

2-Point Discrimination

This simple handheld test is a highly specific evaluation of individual nerve function that can be performed to assess nerve injury and recovery. A 2-point Disk-Criminator is used to determine the shortest distance in millimeters that a patient can appreciate 2 points. This test can be performed in a static or moving mode from distal to proximal in a transverse tip orientation. Normal static values are 6 mm for the index finger and 8 mm for the plantar hallux. Moving values are 2 to 3 mm at the index finger and 4 to 6 mm at the plantar hallux. This test is first performed on the index finger with the patient's eyes open so that they can easily appreciate the test and then with eyes closed for lower extremity testing. The more advanced pressure-specified sensory device is static and moving 2-point discriminator using computer technology to determine sensitivity levels as low as 1 g of pressure (**Fig. 4D–H**).[7]

Vibratory Perception

This test is performed with a metal 2-pronged fork that is an acoustic resonator that produces a perfect sine wave sound pattern. A 128 or 256 Hz (cycles per second) tuning fork are the standard frequency tuning forks used. The delay in seconds counted

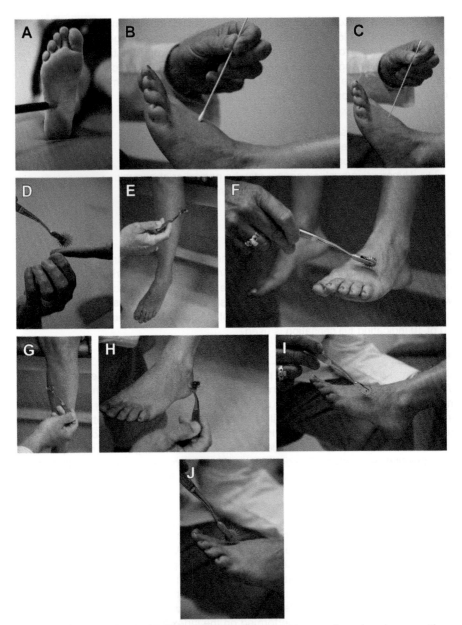

Fig. 3. (*A*) Plantar reflex (Babinski)—L5/S1: Normal—toes down going; absent—no motion; abnormal—toes dorsiflexed. (*B*) Sensory dull testing. (*C*) Sensory sharp testing. (*D*) Index finger sharp testing. (*E*) Common fibular nerve pathway. (*F*) Superficial fibular nerve pathway. (*G*) Saphenous nerve pathway. (*H*) Sural nerve pathway. (*I*) Intermediate dorsal cutaneous nerve pathway. (*J*) Deep fibular nerve pathway.

off between the patient's subjective indication of loss of vibration and the tester's loss of vibration is the basis for this test. The testing pattern is not "nerve specific" as the wave forms penetrate the tissue over a large anatomic area. Areas of individual nerve compression may display heightened sensitivity to this test (**Figs. 4**I, J, **5**A, B).

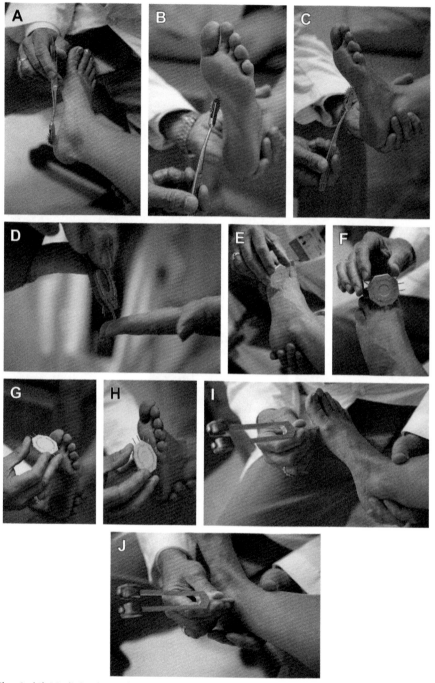

Fig. 4. (*A*) Medial calcaneal nerve pathway. (*B*) Medial plantar nerve pathway. (*C*) Lateral plantar nerve pathway. (*D*) Index finger median nerve. (*E*) Intermediate dorsal cutaneous nerve. (*F*) Deep fibular nerve. (*G*) Medial plantar nerve. (*H*) Lateral plantar nerve. (*I*) Hallux. (*J*) Medial malleolus. (*Courtesy of* [*D–H*] US Neurologicals, LLC, Poulsbo, WA; with permission.)

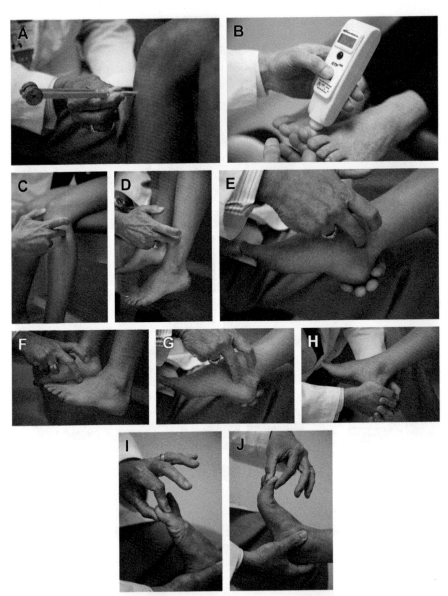

Fig. 5. (*A*) Tibial tubercle. (*B*) Electronic tuning fork: this simple instrument can measure vibratory appreciation in ascending or descending patterns and can average the data to give a more accurate idea of vibratory sensation loss. (*C*) Common fibular nerve. (*D*) Superficial fibular nerve. (*E*) Tibial nerve at the tarsal tunnel. (*F*) Deep fibular nerve. (*G*) Medial/lateral plantar nerves at the port of pedis. (*H*) Medial calcaneal nerve compression test. (*I*) Hallux position down. (*J*) Hallux position up. (*Courtesy of* [*B*] O'Brien Medical, LLC, Orono, ME; with permission.)

Manual Nerve Percussion Test

Percussion of individual peripheral nerve trunks at known sites of fibroosseous tunnels around joints is a valuable diagnostic test that can indicate areas of nerve damage or compression. The Tinel sign is a distally progressing tingling along the course of the nerve indicating an area of nerve regeneration after an injury. The presence of Tinel signs can enable the examiner to map out specific areas of peripheral nerve damage or compression (**Fig. 5C–H**).

Position Sense (Proprioception)

Proprioception is demonstrated in **Fig. 5I, J**.

Additional Testing

Additional testing that can yield useful information is the straight leg test to evaluate sciatic and low back pain, gait examination to assess drop foot conditions, thigh and low back problems, and temperature testing for hot and cold appreciation. Diagnostic peripheral nerve blocks can provide specific information on the anatomic location of pain generators and the relative health of the affected nerve by its reaction to a local anesthetic block. Using small amounts (0.5 mL) of a local anesthetic helps to ensure the specificity of the anesthesia without peripheral geographic anesthetic spread.[8–10]

Summary

The hands-on neurologic examination is the gold standard for developing a working diagnosis for peripheral limb pain. Peripheral nerve trauma, compression neuropathies, metabolic neuropathies, sciatic nerve disorders, low back pathologies, spinal cord diseases, and neurologic pathologies can all be a causative factor in chronic peripheral nerve pain. These simple motor, deep tendon reflex, and sensory examination techniques can rule in or rule out localized diagnoses and provide information possibly indicating a more proximal level of pathology and the need for subsequent referral for additional medical evaluation and diagnostic testing.

In chronic pain syndromes, sensory and motor symptoms can be related to both peripheral and centrally mediated pathologies depending on where the level of injury to the receptor, axon, cell body or intermediate nerve pathway occurs. In the spinal cord, cell bodies of motor nerves are located in the anterior horn and cell bodies of sensory nerves are located in the dorsal root ganglia, for example, light touch, position sense and vibration sense stimuli travel in the spinal cord via the dorsal column system. Sharp, dull, and pain sensation stimuli travel in the spinal cord via the spinothalamic tract. Diminishment or loss of one or more of these senses in a limited geographic area can be owing to specific peripheral nerve lesions at the receptor and nerve trunk level and loss of multiple senses, (traveling in a similar nerve tract), in a larger geographic area may represent a more proximal level of pathology than localized to the legs or feet.

Specific nerve entrapments or areas of injury to a peripheral nerve trunk may demonstrate a mixture of sensory and motor findings. The degree of purely sensory or motor symptoms observed depends on the anatomic level in the limb of the nerve injury and the degree of fascicular arrangement and differentiation in the nerve trunk at the area of injury. Proximal limb injuries can be more mixed sensory and motor in expression and more distal injuries can be more sensory or motor in symptom expression. Anatomically there is more intrafascicular intercommunication proximally in the limb that facilitates mixed sensory and motor findings.

Putting all the pieces of the examination puzzle together in a cogent format can be challenging. It is through the detailed and systematic evaluation of specific nerves, muscles, reflexes, and sensory tests that an accurate working clinical diagnosis can be attained. Prior medical examinations and diagnostic testing may be helpful in ruling out certain diagnoses, but they cannot replace the clinical hands-on assessment of the patient.

REFERENCES

1. Dellon AL. Somatosensory testing and rehabilitation. Rockville (MD): American Association of Hand Therapy; 1997. Chapter 7.
2. Barrett SL. Pain and presurgical screening. In: Barrett SL, editor. Practical pain management for the lower extremity surgeon. 1st edition. Brooklandville (MD): Data Trace Publishing Company; 2015. p. 103–11.
3. Zatouroff M, Bouffler LE. The foot in neurological disease. In: Bouffler LE, editor. A colour atlas of the foot in clinical diagnosis. 1st edition. Aylesbury (United Kingdom): Hazell Books; 1992. p. 201–15.
4. Saraffian SK, Kelikian AS. Nerves. In: Kelikian AS, editor. Anatomy of the foot and ankle. 3rd edition. Philadelphia: Lippincott Williams and Wilkins; 2011. p. 381–427.
5. Adelaar RS. Peripheral nerve disorders of the foot and ankle. In: Sammarco GJ, Cooper PS, editors. Foot and ankle manual. 2nd edition. Baltimore: Williams and Wilkins; 1998. p. 321–39.
6. Cailliet R. Neurologic examination. In: Cailliet R, editor. Foot and ankle pain. Philadelphia: F. A. Davis Co; 1997. p. 89–91.
7. Seiler D, Wilton J, Dellon A. Detection of neuropathy due to mycobacterium leprae using noninvasive neurosensory testing of susceptible peripheral nerves. Ann Plast Surg 2005;55:633.
8. Barrett SL. Practical neurologic examination and understanding the performance of diagnostic nerve blocks. In: Barrett SL, editor. Practical pain management for the lower extremity surgeon. 1st edition. Brooklandville (MD): Data Trace Publishing Company; 2015. p. 91–103.
9. Sardesai AM, Logan BM. Regional anesthesia. In: Sardesai AM, editor. McMinn's color atlas of foot and ankle anatomy. 4th edition. Philadelphia: WB Saunders; 2012. p. 125–31.
10. Logan BM. Muscles and nerves of the lower extremity. In: Logan BM, editor. McMinn's color atlas of foot and ankle anatomy. 4th edition. Philadelphia: WB Saunders; 2012. p. 116–23.

Multiple Crush Concept Applied to Multiple Nerves in Leprous Neuropathy

A. Lee Dellon, MD, PhD*

KEYWORDS

- Leprosy • Neurolysis • Nerve compression

KEY POINTS

- A Norwegian doctor, Gerhard Henrik Armauer Hansen, in 1873, found that leprosy was caused by a bacteria. *Mycobacterium leprae* is mildly contagious and does not pass through the skin. It is inhaled.
- An orthopedic surgeon, Paul Brand, in Vellore, India, in 1948, identified a neural origin of leprous deformity and refuted the dissolving flesh theory of leprosy.
- The World Health Organization introduced multidrug therapy in 1981: it stops leprosy spread but does not decrease disability related to its chronic nerve injury.
- An adhesion molecule was identified in 1997 that links the *M leprae* to the G domain of laminin and the Schwann cell.
- In 2004, James Wilton, DPM, and A. Lee Dellon, MD, first applied the concept of decompression of multiple sites of neurolysis along individual nerves in the upper and lower extremities to patients with leprous neuritis.

INTRODUCTION

And the leper in whom the plaque is, his clothes shall be rent, and his head bare, and he shall put a covering upon his upper lip, and shall cry, Unclean, unclean. All the days wherein the plaque shall be in him he shall be defiled; he is unclean; he shall dwell alone; without the camp shall his habitation be.

—Leviticus 13.45–46

It is most likely that doctors reading this article will never have seen even 1 person with leprosy. What is leprosy? The very first definition of it was given by God to Aaron, the brother of Moses, and it is recorded in dermatologic fashion in Leviticus 13.1–46. The date of this recording and clinical observations are, of course unknown. It seems

Johns Hopkins University, Baltimore, MD, USA
* 1122 Kenilworth Drive, Suite 18, Towson, MD 21204.
E-mail address: aldellon@dellon.com

Clin Podiatr Med Surg 33 (2016) 203–217
http://dx.doi.org/10.1016/j.cpm.2015.12.009
0891-8422/16/$ – see front matter © 2016 Elsevier Inc. All rights reserved.

clear, however, that leprosy was considered infectious. In 1841, Gerhard Henrik Armauer Hansen was born in Bergen, Norway. Bergen was the center of Norwegian leprosy research and there were 3000 lepers in Bergen, 800 hospitalized. After medical school, Hansen, after observing these patients, did not believe the prevailing theory that the disease was inherited. Traveling in Europe, he studied the emerging science of histopathology and tissue staining. No human disease had yet been proved to be transmitted by a bacteria. When Hansen returned to Bergen in 1871, he identified rodlike structures in cells of cutaneous nodules and published his article in 1873 describing *M leprae*.[1,2] Leprosy today is known as Hansen disease. Hansen was unable to get this disease to be transmitted from one animal to another or one human to another, and therefore failed to satisfy Koch's postulates that proved a disease was due to a bacteria. Yet this recognition within Norway led to legislation in 1877 and 1885, the Leprosy Acts that permitted lepers to live apart from their families, in precautionary isolation, resulting in the decrease in incidence of leprosy in Norway (**Fig. 1**).

The first use of antibiotics for "treatment" of leprosy was done by Robert Greenhill Cochrane, MD (1899–1985), a Scottish dermatologist, working in India in a leprosy "sanatorium" in Chingleput, in the southeast of the country. He also worked in Vellore, just north of Chennai (Madras). Dapsone, a sulfur derivative, was administered intramuscularly in oil and was bacteriostatic. This became the main treatment for the next 30 years for leprosy. Cochrane would write 3 books on leprosy from 1947 to 1964.[3–5]

Cochrane had a direct impact on the current approach to leprosy by inducing Paul Wilson Brand, MD (1914–2003), to come and work in Vellore. Cochrane knew Brand's parents, who had been Christian missionaries in India, where Brand was born in 1914. When World War II ended, Brand had just finished orthopedic surgery training in the United Kingdom. His wife Margaret was an ophthalmologist. Although Cochrane described in great detail the dermatologic consequences of leprosy, Brand was struck

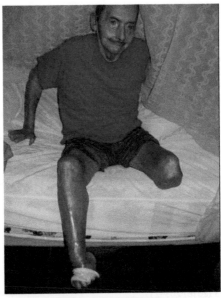

Fig. 1. Typical appearance of extremities with amputations in a person with leprosy who has not had peripheral nerve surgery. This person is living in a sanctuary in Ecuador.

by the upper extremity and lower extremity deformities. He recalled as a child in India seeing children with bones protruding from their feet but them not having any pain. As a medical student he had dissected cranial nerves and was amazed at the facial palsy present in the lepers. Charles Scott Sherrington (1857–1952), one of his teachers, a professor of physiology at the University of Oxford, went on to win the Nobel prize in 1932 for his work in neurophysiology. This exposure to Sherrington's peripheral nerve research fascinated Brand, and he pondered the relationship between leprosy and the peripheral nerve. Brand reviewed the orthopedic literature at that time and found that nothing had been written about leprosy.[6]

The religion of the population in Vellore was Hindu, and, therefore, Brand did not have the ability to do autopsies on people with leprosy. Brand noted,

> ...frequent paralysis in areas controlled by the ulnar nerve (**Fig. 2A**), moderate paralysis in median nerve, and very little in the radial nerve. I could think of no logical reason why the ulnar nerve at the elbow would cause paralysis while the median nerve, one inch away, stayed healthy; or why the median nerve went dead at the wrist while none of the radial nerve muscles was paralyzed. To add to my confusion, I had sent tissue samples from shortened fingers to Vellore's pathology professor (**Fig. 2B**). The reports came back as normal tissue, except for the loss of nerve endings.[6]

One night, in a somewhat distant forest village, a leprosy patient without relatives died, and word of this came to Brand and his team. They were able to travel through the night and complete the removal of peripheral nerves from the arms and legs of that person. Brandt wrote,

> On one side of the body, sections of the nerves were put into bottles and labeled, on the other side I dissected out the entire length of the nerves: I wanted to see the whole nerve in relation to the bones and muscles.... When I stood and looked, finally taking a break, I saw it. 'Look at the nerve swellings. Do you see a pattern?' At certain places, behind the ankle, just above the knee, and also at the wrist, the nerves swelled up to many times normal size...and were most marked just above the elbow on the ulnar nerve (**Fig. 3**)....We saw clearly that nerve swellings tended to occur in just a few sites... where the nerve lay close to the skin surface, and not in the deep tissues. For the first time I sensed some rationality behind the mystery of leprosy-induced paralysis.[6]

Brand (**Fig. 4**) went on to develop the concept of tendon transfers to provide function for the loss of the muscles lost to superficial nerve injury from leprosy by replacement with the "preserved" deeper muscles whose nerves were not injured by the leprosy bacteria. He published continually on this work from 1952 through 1989.[7–18]

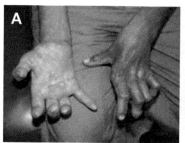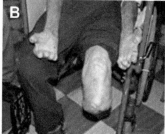

Fig. 2. Typical appearance of progressive neurologic deformity that results in (*A*) clawing and amputation in the upper extremity and (*B*) amputation in the lower extremity.

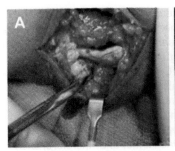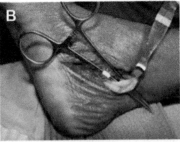

Fig. 3. Brand's observations about the swelling in the major superficial nerves just proximal to a joint are illustrated here from our own experience in Ecuador. (*A*) The swollen ulnar nerve just proximal to the elbow. (*B*) The swollen tibial nerve just proximal to the ankle.

When Brand opened the Raymond M. Curtis Hand Center in Baltimore in 1977, it was the year that I was doing my hand surgery fellowship and focusing on peripheral nerve problems.

DRUG THERAPY DOES NOT PREVENT NEUROLOGIC IMPAIRMENT

Drug therapy stops contagion. The purpose of controlling leprosy, however, must include a reduction in the rate and severity of disability. The key to effective management of leprosy is early diagnosis and drug treatment and early recognition and management of nerve damage, combined with effective health education.

Leprosy is an infectious disease but it has many features in common with neurodegenerative disorders. It results in a chronic neurologic illness, which is progressive unless treated; frequently, it produces long-term disability and is associated with high levels of stigma (missing digits, facial disfigurement, and skin color changes).

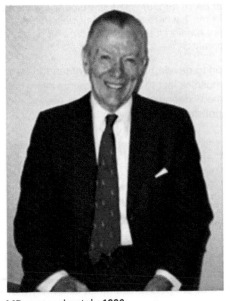

Fig. 4. Paul W. Brand, MD, approximately 1990.

As leprosy has a known infective agent, *M leprae*, there is the possibility of disease control. Multidrug treatment with the antibiotic combination rifampicin, dapsone, and clofazimine is highly effective in curing infection, with relapse rates of 1%.[19] It was hoped that having effective antibiotics would permit disease control and thus the concept of "leprosy elimination" developed. "Leprosy elimination by the year 2000" was first proposed in 1986 and at the 44th World Health Assembly in 1991 modified by the addendum "as a public health problem," defined as less than 1 case per 10,000 population.[20] Many patients experience immune-mediated nerve damage, which may occur before, during, or after treatment. Field-based cohort studies have shown that at diagnosis of leprosy, at the start of multidrug therapy, many patients already have established nerve damage; rates vary from 20% in Bangladesh to 56% in Ethiopia,[21,22] and these patients have a worse prognosis for disability. Anesthesia and paresis in the hands and feet put leprosy patients at risk of secondary damage from trauma and infection, which cause the highly visible deformities of leprosy.

Despite multidrug therapy, in 2005 there were 500,000 new cases of leprosy in the world per year, 12% of which in children, and 200 of which in the United States: there were 12 million lepers in the World and 6000 were in the United States.[23–25]

When Brand retired from his work in India, he became the Director of the National Leprosarium of the United States, in Carville, Louisiana. There he used a form of quantitative sensory testing with the Semmes-Weinstein monofilaments to document sensibility in many different areas of the hand and foot. He remained unenthusiastic about nerve decompression surgery in patients with leprosy.[18]

HISTORY OF PERIPHERAL NERVE SURGERY IN LEPROSY

There is a small body of literature related to peripheral nerve surgery in leprosy. A few studies of nerve grafting for irreparable damage to the ulnar nerve, usually in the presence of abscess, were reported in the late 1970s. Nerve graft results did not give improved function.[26–28]

There are many more reports of decompression of the ulnar nerve at the elbow for the treatment of pain, utilizing the whole spectrum of reported procedures with the exception of submuscular transposition.[29–35] In general these studies have reported significant pain relief, with some improvement in sensation and some improvement in motor function. The claim is made that deformity is prevented when the nerve decompression is done in early cases. It is noted the electrophysiological tests do not recover to more than 80% of normal function, and often much less, even when there is good clinical and symptomatic improvement.[35] Much less has been written about carpal tunnel decompression for the median nerve. In the 1 article devoted just to this nerve, of 29 patients who had a decompression, sensory recovery was seen in 90% of cases, and in 45% muscle strength improved, whereas in another 25% motor function had no further detioration.[35]

Median nerve decompression is also commented on in 1 of the studies reporting ulnar nerve results.[34] Where the degree of nerve compression was graded preoperatively and clinically staged, of 3 patients with moderate degree of compression, only 1 patient improved, and 2 had no change, in contrast to 6 patients with severe compression, of whom 3 recovered normal strength and improved sensation, 2 cases were worse, and 1 was not improved. When median nerve postoperative results are compared with those after cubital tunnel decompression using this same staging paradigm, for the moderate degree of ulnar nerve compression, of 15 patients, 4 were better and 11 were not improved. For the severe degree of compression, of 17 patients, 6 were better, 5 were without change, and 6 were worse.[35] Results from

Husain and colleagues[34] for the ulnar decompression were also in the same area of success, although they did not clinically stage their patients' degree of compression; although 49% had relief of pain, 11% failed to improve in terms of sensory or motor recovery, and those who had some degree of improvement were combined with those who "were prevented from getting worse to give the appearance that 89% of patients were benefited by the ulnar nerve surgery."

Pandya's[30] report, in addition to including carpal and cubital tunnel decompression, included tarsal tunnel decompression and neurolysis of the common peroneal nerve. There are 3 other brief reports on tarsal tunnel surgery. One, using sweat production as a functional outcome measure, reported an improvement after a traditional posterior tibial nerve decompression[36]; the second added an internal neurolysis of the posterior tibial nerve and a sympathectomy to restore sensation and improve ulcer healing in a single patient[37]; and the third, written in French in 1976, suggests a role for neurolysis of the tibial nerve in patients with leprosy and diabetes.[38]

Past approaches to nerve decompression have applied the concept of decompressing 1 nerve in 1 location at 1 operation, or, at most, 2 different nerves were decompressed, each at 1 location along the course of the nerve.

With regard to Brand's indication for peripheral nerve surgery requiring a course of steroids, it is interesting to look at 2 of the most scientifically designed studies related to the treatment of peripheral nerve problems in leprosy. In 1996, for the treatment of "early ulnar neuritis," a randomized trial of ulnar neurolysis combined with medial epicondylectomy was compared with a full course of high-dose steroids. There were approximately 20 patients in each group, and they were followed for 2 years. There was no difference in the outcomes between the 2 groups.[39] In 2003, a multicentered, randomized, double-blind, placebo-controlled trial was conducted in Nepal and Bangladesh, with 1 group getting either high-dose prednisolone, tapered over 4 months, and 1 group receiving a placebo. In this study, patients had a higher degree of nerve function impairment (NFI) then in the previous study, with duration of NFI ranging from 6 to 24 months. Of 92 patients followed for 1 year, "no demonstrable additional improvement in nerve function, or in preventing further leprosy reaction events was seen in the prednisolone group. Overall, improvement of nerve function at 12 months was seen in about 50% of patients in both groups. This result was the same for the ulnar nerve and for the posterior tibial nerve. Leprosy reactions and new NFI occurred in a third of the group, emphasizing the need to keep patients under regular surveillance during multidrug therapy, and, where possible, after completion of multidrug therapy."[40]

Summarizing the diverse, retrospective case studies in the surgical literature on leprosy from the past 25 years, it can only be inferred that traditional decompression surgery can relieve pain often, improve function in less than 50%, and have the potential to result in even worse peripheral nerve function. With regard to the only 2 high-level evidence-based studies, it could be summarized by saying that for the ulnar nerve at the elbow, steroids gave no better results than surgery, and steroids gave no better results than doing nothing; therefore, by inference, there is no demonstrated value in doing surgery in terms of functional improvement.

A NEW CONCEPTUAL APPROACH TO NEUROLYSIS IN LEPROSY

In 2002, as I read Brand and Yancey's book about pain, *The Gift Nobody Wants*,[6] I realized that his clinical investigative journey, concluding that peripheral nerves were the cause of the leprosy disability and noting the swelling of nerves proximal to a known anatomic site of compression, was similar to my journey trying to help patients with progressive neurologic problems related to neuropathy, especially diabetic neuropathy. I concluded that much of the disability, termed *diabetic peripheral neuropathy*, was due to the presence of multiple nerve compressions along the course of individual nerves.[41–43] The surgical solution to this puzzle was to decompress multiple sites along the course of each peripheral nerve, and this resulted in relief of pain, recovery of sensation, and, consequent to this, prevention of ulceration and amputation.[44]

Would the surgical approaches developed to restore sensation and prevent ulceration and amputation in diabetics with neuropathy and nerve compression be able to help patients with leprosy and nerve compression? These approaches were based on the double crush concept that multiple sites of compression might need to be decompressed simultaneously along the course of an individual peripheral nerve.

To evaluate this, I began work in Guayaquil, Ecuador, with Wilton, a podiatric foot and ankle surgeon, from Portsmouth, New Hampshire, because he had been providing club foot care in Ecuador with the Perfect World Foundation. A team was formed to evaluate approximately 40 people at the Father Damien house in Guayaquil. The Father Damien House residents had received triple antibiotic therapy for their *M leprae* and were no longer contagious, although they still became progressively more disabled due to what is now understood to be their peripheral nerve problems. Seiler did neurosensory testing with the pressure-specified sensory device (**Table 1**), and Wilton identified nerve entrapments by a positive Tinel sign. **Fig. 5** shows 2 patients not chosen to be candidates for surgery and **Fig. 6** shows a patient chosen for nerve decompression by that team.

Then, in September of 2004, Dellon and Wilton, with the operating nurses and anesthesiology team that Wilton organized, went back to Guayaquil and operated simultaneously on upper and lower extremities of 20 patients chosen by the first team (**Fig. 7**).

Given that excellent surgeons had attempted to decompress nerves in patients with leprosy in the past, what could we add to improve the chance of success? The double crush concept applied to leprosy suggested that the host response to *M leprae* occurred at locations where the nerve was superficial and where there were known sites of nerve compression. The conclusion was to decompress each nerve at each site in which it could be decompressed in that extremity. For the ulnar nerve, the decompression had to be at the elbow and at the wrist, and the decompression at the wrist had to include the motor branch of the ulnar nerve (**Fig. 8**). For the median nerve, the decompression had to be the wrist and also, if possible, in the forearm. In the absence of specifically finding evidence of the pronator syndrome, the approach

Table 1
Leprosy in Ecuador: neurosensory testing. Distribution of peripheral nerves evaluated with the pressure-specified sensory device

Peripheral Nerve	Number of Nerves Tested
Median	29
Ulnar	40
Radial sensory	2
Peroneal	30
Tibial	18
Sural	1
Total	120

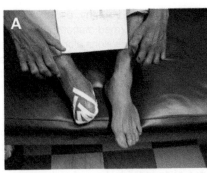
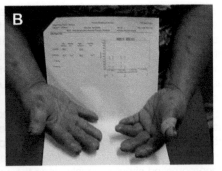

Fig. 5. Two patients whose degrees of paralysis, amputation, and sensory loss were too advanced to be included for surgery. (*A*) Note amputated fingers. (*B*) Note neurosensory testing with the pressure-specified sensory device demonstrated absent static 2-point discrimination and even 1-point discrimination. Neither of these patients had a positive Tinel sign.

used to the ulnar nerve decompression, the submuscular transposition by the musculofascial lengthening technique, demonstrating the best long-term results, would decompress the median nerve at the elbow by lengthening the superficial head of the pronator and incising the lacertus fibrosus (**Fig. 9**).

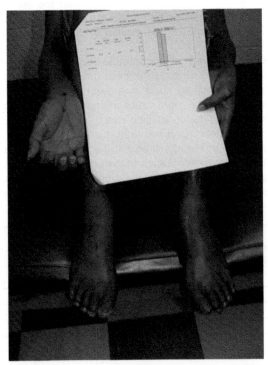

Fig. 6. This patient had neurosensory testing consistent with moderate degree of nerve compression and had a positive Tinel sign. Therefore, this patient was a candidate for nerve decompression.

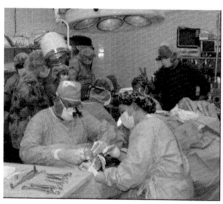

Fig. 7. Operating room organization for 2-team approach to nerve decompression in patient with leprosy. Doctor with hand up indicating V for victory is the anesthesiologist at the head of the operating table. Wilton, foreground, is operating on the right leg, and Dellon, back of head to camera, in center of photograph, is operating on the right arm.

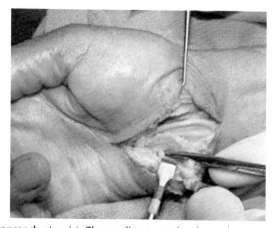

Fig. 8. Surgical approach at wrist. The median nerve has been decompressed in the carpal tunnel and Guyon canal is opened to decompress the ulnar nerve. Clamp demonstrates the hypertrophic ulnar motor branch after incising the hypothenar muscle fascia at the hook of the hamate.

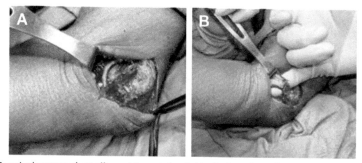

Fig. 9. Surgical approach at elbow. Musculofascial technique for submuscular transposition of ulnar nerve at elbow shows (A) the muscle flaps that have been created, with ulnar nerve lying above, on muscle, and (B) muscle flaps transposed and lengthened, permitting finger and ulnar nerve to lie beneath. This approach also decompresses the proximal median nerve.

The radial nerve at the elbow lies deep to muscles and would likely not be invaded by *M leprae*, but superficial sensory branch should be decompressed in the forearm (**Fig. 10**).

For the tibial nerve, its branches in the medial and lateral plantar and calcaneal tunnels are decompressed (**Fig. 11**).

For the peroneal nerve, it would be decompressed at both the fibular neck and over the dorsum of the foot and, if there were a positive Tinel sign, over the superficial peroneal nerve in the leg.

Internal neurolysis was done as indicated, based on intraoperative findings of firmness, intraneural fibrosis, and loss of perineurial markings (**Fig. 12**).

RESULTS IN THE EARLY SERIES OF PATIENTS

Twelve patients had the surgical approach shown in **Table 2**, with surgical decompression of 3 nerves in an arm and 3 nerves in a leg done simultaneously. They each received intravenous cephalosporin prior to inflating the tourniquets, and they continued oral cephalosporin for 1 week postoperatively. There were no surgical complications. There were no anesthesia complications. As indicated from **Table 2**, there was a wide range of impairment preoperatively in these patients. They were each kept the first night in the hospital and were returned to the Father Damien House the day after the surgery. On examining them the day after surgery, many who did not have fixed joint deformities in the hand (clawing) could already straighten their fingers and make a better fist. One patient is shown as an example of early recovery of sensibility in the foot after extensive neurolysis of the posterior tibial nerve and its branches (**Fig. 13**) and another as an example of early recovery of motor function (**Fig. 14**).

The mid-November 2004, 2-month follow-up was remarkable for no wound infections. Two patients who lived far away were not back for follow-up. Of the remaining 10 patients, 7 said they had better sensation in the hand and foot that were operated on than they had before surgery, and they had better feeling in these operated extremities than they did in the nonoperated extremities. Three patients noted no improvement. No patient was worse. The results were recorded by Dr Martinez and submitted by e-mail in the form of a chart for each patient by e-mail.

A 1-year follow-up mission returned in 2005, led by Wilton and Scott Nickerson, an orthopedic surgeon not involved in the initial surgery; they went to do the

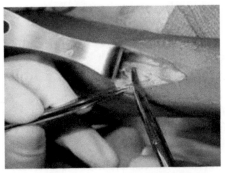

Fig. 10. Surgical approach to radial nerve in forearm. Fascia has been divided. Hand is to the right, and elbow is to the left. Note proximal normal size of nerve, and distally, at exit from fascia, there is enlargement of nerve at site of entrapment.

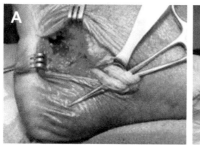
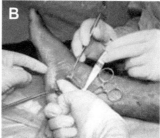

Fig. 11. Surgical approach to the tibial nerve at the ankle. (A) After releasing the tarsal tunnel itself, an internal neurolysis of medial and lateral plantar nerves was done because of the presence of intraneural fibrosis. (B) After release of the medial and lateral plantar tunnels and excision of septum between medial and lateral plantar tunnels to create 1 large tunnel, note that surgeon's finger extends into the plantar aspect of the foot.

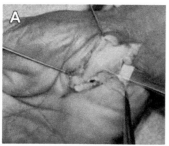
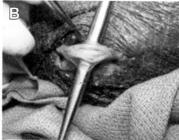

Fig. 12. Examples of internal neurolysis in upper extremity. (A) Excision of epineurium and intraneural neurolysis of median nerve at wrist. (B) Excision of epineurium and intraneural neurolysis of the ulnar nerve at elbow.

Table 2
Documentation and staging of peripheral nerve dysfunction with the pressure-specified sensory device

	Grading of Degree of Sensory Nerve Compression		
Peripheral Nerve	(Mild–Moderate)	(Severe)	(Anesthetic)
Median	41%	24%	35%
Ulnar	35%	37%	28%
Peroneal	10%	13%	77%
Tibial	11%	16%	73%

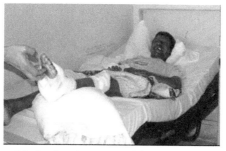

Fig. 13. Patient smiling while having the operated foot tickled, indicating improved sensation 1 day (24 hours) after neurolysis of the tibial nerve and its branches in the 4 medial ankle tunnels. He had severe sensory loss prior to surgery.

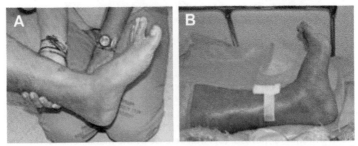

Fig. 14. Patient with improved motor function 24 hours after having neurolysis of the common peroneal nerve at the knee. (*A*) immediately preoperatively, inability to extend big toe and dorsiflex ankle; (*B*) immediately postoperatively, after neurolysis of common peroneal nerve at the knee, note ability now to extend big toe and dorsiflex the ankle.

postoperative physical examinations. Postoperative neurosensory testing was also done. Overall, of the 12 patients operated on, 6 were in the excellent category (**Fig. 15**) and 4 were in the good category, with only 2 patients not improved. No one was worse. The entire follow-up team is noted in **Fig. 16**.

Subsequent missions have accounted for approximately 150 patients having had approximately 700 nerve surgeries. Future challenges include designing a prospective

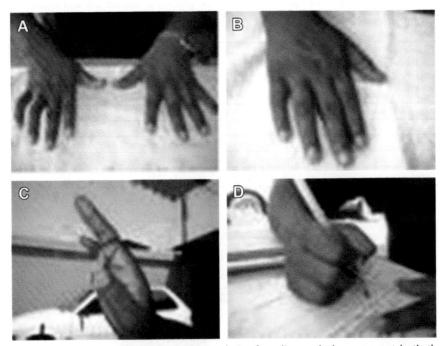

Fig. 15. Improved hand function after neurolysis of median and ulnar nerve at both the wrist and elbow regions. (*A*) Preoperatively, note clawing and wasting of first dorsal interosseous muscle. Postoperatively at 1-year follow-up, note (*B*) reversal of clawing, (*C*) ability to pinch, and (*D*) ability to write.

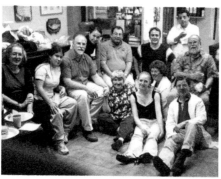

Fig. 16. In 2005, a team returned to Ecuador to do a 1-year evaluation of the first group of leprosy patients to have this surgery. Seated on the floor, from the left are Sister Annie Credidio, BVM, Damien House Director; Shannon Wilton and Rosemary Wayes, who did neurosensory testing for Wilton; and David Seiler, MBA, who did the neurosensory testing for Dellon. In the second row, seated, are Anne Nickerson, a local host; James Wilton, who led the team; a local host, Dale Montgomery, from the Perfect World Foundation, which sponsored the team; and David Nickerson and his father Scott Nickerson, MD, an orthopedic surgeon, who, uninvolved in the first surgery itself, did the postoperative physical examinations. Martinez is the physician at the Damien House. Standing in the third row is Martinez, the Damien House physician. Shannon Wilton and Anne and David Nickerson served as translators.

study with appropriate outcomes and implementation of this surgical strategy on a worldwide scale.

REFERENCES

1. Available at: www.telecom.net.et/ahri/hansen.html.
2. Available at: www.whonamedit.com/doctor.cfm/596.html.
3. Cochrane RG. Practical textbook of leprosy. London: G. Cumberlege Pub; 1947.
4. Cochrane RG. Biblical leprosy: a suggested interpretation. London: Tyndale Press; 1963.
5. Cochrane RB, Davey TF, editors. Leprosy in theory and practice. Bristol (England): Wright and Sons; 1964.
6. Brand P, Yancey P. The gift nobody wants. New York: Harper; 1995.
7. Brand PW. The orthopedic care of leprosy patients. Lepr Rev 1952;23:50–62.
8. Brand PW. The reconstruction of the hand in leprosy. Ann R Coll Surg Engl 1952; 11:350–61.
9. Brand PW. The place of physical medicine and orthopedic surgery in leprosy. Lepr Rev 1954;25:5–10.
10. Brand PW. Treatment of leprosy II. The role of surgery. N Engl J Med 1956;254: 64–7.
11. Brand PW. Paralytic claw hand; with special reference to paralysis in leprosy and treatment by sublimis transfer Stiles and Bunnell. J Bone Joint Surg 1958;40B: 618–32.
12. Brand PW. Temperature variation and leprosy deformity. Int J Lepr 1959;27:1–7.
13. Brand PW. Life after leprosy though rehabilitation. Rehabil Lit 1960;21:239–45.
14. Bauman JH, Girling JP, Brand PW. Plantar pressures and trophic ulceration. An evaluation of foot wear. J Bone Joint Surg 1963;4B:652–73.

15. Harris JR, Brand PW. Pattern of disintegration of the tarsus in the anesthetic foot. J Bone Joint Surg 1964;48B:4–16.

16. Edgerton MT, Brand PW. Restoration of abduction and adduction to the unstable thumb in median and ulnar paralysis. Plast Reconstr Surg 1965;36:150–64.

17. Hastings RC, Brand PW, Mansfield RE, et al. Bacterial density in the skin in lepromatous leprosy as related to temperature. Lepr Rev 1968;39:71–4.

18. Brand PW, Fritschi EP. Rehabilitation in leprosy. In: Hastings RC, editor. Leprosy. 1st edition. London: Chruchill Livingstone; 1985. p. 287–319.

19. WHO Expert Committee on Leprosy. Seventh report. World Health Organ Tech Rep Ser 1998;874:20.

20. World Health Assembly. Elimination of leprosy: resolution of the 44th World Health Assembly. Geneva (Switzerland): World Health Organization; 1991 (Resolution No WHA 44.9).

21. Saunderson P, Gebre S, Desta K, et al. The pattern of leprosy-related neuropathy in the AMFES patients in Ethiopia: definitions, incidence, risk factors and outcome. Lepr Rev 2000;71:285–308.

22. Croft RP, Nicholls PG, Richardus JH, et al. The treatment of acute nerve function impairment in leprosy: results from a prospective cohort study in Bangladesh. Lepr Rev 2000;71:154–68.

23. Available at: www.eneducube,cin/derm/topic223.html.

24. Available at: www.hhmi.org/bioactive/disease/leprosy/. Accessed February 5, 2005.

25. CDC. MMWR 2003;50(53). Available at: www.cdc.goc.html.

26. Anon N. Nerve grafts in leprosy. Lancet 1975;2:216–7.

27. McLeod JG, Hargrave JC, Gye RS, et al. Nerve grafting in leprosy. Brain 1975;98:203–12.

28. Miko TL. Nerve grafting in Leprosy. Lancet 1993;342:1429.

29. Palande DD. A review of twenty-three operations on the ulnar nerve in leprous neuritis. J Bone Joint Surg 1973;55A:1457–64.

30. Pandya NJ. Surgical decompression of nerves in leprosy. An attempt at prevention of deformities. A clinical, electrophysiologic, histopathologic and surgical study. Int J Lepr Other Mycobact Dis 1978;46:47–55.

31. Malaviya GN, Ramu G. Role of surgical decompression in ulnar neuritis of leprosy. Lepr India 1982;54:287–302.

32. Ramarorazana S, DiSchino M, Rene JP, et al. Results of 466 nerve decompressions in 123 leprosy patients during polychemotherapy with a minimum follow-up of one year. Value of preventive surgery in a leprosy control program. Arch Inst Pasteur Madagascar 1994;61:115–7.

33. Husain S, Mishra B, Prakash V, et al. Results of surgical decompression of ulnar nerve in leprosy. Acta Leprol 1998;11:17–20.

34. Husain S, Kumar A, Yadav VS, et al. Ulnar and median nerves in paucibacillary leprosy; a follow-up study of electrophysiological function in patients before and after nerve trunk decompression. Lepr Rev 2003;74:374–82.

35. Husain S, Mishra B, Prakash V, et al. Evaluation of the surgical decompression of median nerve in leprosy in relation to sensory and motor functions. Acta Leprol 1997;10:199–201.

36. Oommen PK. Posterior tibial neurovascular decompression for restoration of plantar sweating and sensibility. Indian J Lepr 1996;68:75–82.

37. de Coninck A, Helou S, Bins EJ. Perforating plantar ulcer. Interfascicular neurolysis for the posterior tibial nerve. Sem Hop 1983;16:1823–6.

38. Bourel P, Rey A, Blanc JF, et al. Tarsal tunnel syndrome; 15 "pure" cases and 100 cases "combined with leprosy or diabetes. Rev Rhum Mal Osteoartic 1976;43: 723–8.
39. Ebenezer M, Andrews P, Solomon S. Comparative trial of steroids and surgical intervention in the management of ulnar neuritis. Int J Lepr Other Mycobact Dis 1996;64:282–6.
40. Richardus JH, Withington SG, Anderson AM, et al. Treatment with corticosteroids of long-standing nerve function impairment in leprosy: a randomized controlled trial. Lepr Rev 2003;74:311–8.
41. Dellon ES, Dellon AL, Seiler WA IV. The effect of tarsal tunnel decompression in the streptozotocin-induced diabetic rat. Microsurg 1994;15:265–8.
42. Aszmann OC, Tassler PL, Dellon AL. Changing the natural history of diabetic neuropathy: incidence of ulcer/amputation in the contralateral limb of patients with a unilateral nerve decompression procedure. Ann Plast Surg 2004;53:517–22.
43. Dellon AL. The dellon approach to neurolysis in the neuropathy patient with chronic nerve compression. Handchir Mikrochir Plast Chir 2008;40:1–10.
44. Dellon AL, Muse VL, Nickerson DS. Prevention of ulceration, amputation and reduction of hospitalization: outcomes of a prospective multi-center trial of tibial neurolysis in patients with diabetic neuropathy. J Reconstr Microsurg 2012;28: 241–6.

Chronic Exertional Compartment Syndrome

 CrossMark

Richard T. Braver, DPM*

KEYWORDS

- Chronic exertional compartment syndrome • Chronic compartment syndrome
- Intracompartmental pressure testing • Fasciotomy • Exercise induced leg pain
- Medial tibial stress syndrome • Shin splints • Soleus bridge • Exercise neuropraxia

KEY POINTS

- Increased tissue pressure within a fascial compartment may be the result from any increase in volume within its contents or any decrease in size of the fascial covering or due to any distensibility of the fascial covering (ie, patients with thickened fascia).
- Shin splint pain and chronic exertional compartment syndrome (CECS) can be differentiated by a careful history and by exclusion of other maladies and confirmed by compartmental syndrome testing.
- Once the practitioner makes the proper diagnoses of CECS, through clinical examination and intracompartmental testing, surgical fasciotomy along with ancillary procedures should allow the athlete to return to competitive activity.

Patients who experience intense pain, a burning sensation, tightness, and/or numbness in the lower extremities during exercise activity, whereby the pain resolves quickly after cessation of activity, can often be diagnosed with chronic exertional compartment syndrome (CECS). This syndrome was first described by Mavor[1] in 1956 in which there was increased pressure within a specific muscle compartment of the leg, which causes pressure on vessels and nerves causing the symptoms.

Mubarak and Hargens[2] studied *acute* compartment syndrome (not to be confused with CECS) that included decreased blood flow through the intracompartmental capillaries (capillary ischemia), but continued blood flow to larger arteries and veins with palpable pulses distally.

In a study performed with magnetic resonance imaging, Amendola and colleagues[3] found that CECS is not related to ischemia, but is actually due to increased fluid content within the muscle compartment. This can compromise or impair function of the muscles or nerves within a tight and constricted fascial covering.

It is also hypothesized by myself, as well as several colleagues, that the symptoms of CECS are similar to those individuals diagnosed with lumbar spinal stenosis who

Department of Podiatry, Hackensack University Medical Center, Hackensack, NJ, USA
* Corresponding author. c/o Active Foot & Ankle Care, LLC, 4-14 Saddle River Road, Suite 101, Fair Lawn, NJ 07410.
E-mail address: DrRun@aol.com

Clin Podiatr Med Surg 33 (2016) 219–233
http://dx.doi.org/10.1016/j.cpm.2015.12.002
0891-8422/16/$ – see front matter © 2016 Elsevier Inc. All rights reserved.

experience pain, weakness, and numbness causing them to limp. Like spinal stenosis, CECS may be the result of "temporary neurogenic claudication." Here the small capillaries that supply the leg nerves are not getting their normal blood supply because they are compressed by increased compartment content during exercise.

In addition, several colleagues and I think that in CECS, nerve(s) and its pain receptors, such as mechanoreceptors and nociceptors are stimulated by any increased abnormal pressure against them.

Detmer and colleagues[4] found in their study of 100 patients that most cases of CECS involve both legs, although other studies have indicated 80% or more involve both legs. It should also be noted in the study by Detmer and colleagues[4] that the condition affected men and women pretty equally. In my private practice working with several universities and running clubs, I would concur with these findings and note that our average patient with CECS is a competitive athlete between the ages of 18 and 25. We have found equal occurrence among sprint sport athletes as in long distance runners.

Other physical findings of CECS may include mild edema or muscle herniations over the involved compartment, and muscle weakness of a specific compartment. This may include weakness of: dorsiflexion (anterior compartment), eversion/abduction (lateral compartment), plantar flexion (superficial posterior compartment), or inversion/toe flexion (deep posterior compartment).

Symptoms present during exercise also may include paresthesia to the anterior leg or ankle, or between the first and second metatarsal due to involvement of the medial terminal branch of the deep peroneal nerve within the anterior compartment.

If the patient complains of numbness or tingling to the arch or plantar aspect of the foot during exercise activity, that may be associated with a deep posterior leg compartment syndrome and not just a tarsal tunnel syndrome. In my personal experience, however, most patients do not complain of numbness, rather they complain of pain and tightness, which most often forces the athlete to curtail his or her activity level or stop to rest.

DIFFERENTIAL DIAGNOSES

The diagnosis of CECS is initially a diagnosis made by exclusion. Later on it is confirmed by intracompartmental pressure testing.

Often times, the deep posterior muscle compartments may have symptoms of medial tibial stress syndrome or chronic shin splints. Standard treatment of nonsteroidal anti-inflammatory drugs, orthotics, shin splint taping, rehabilitation, and so forth, should be initiated. The practitioner must be keenly aware of biomechanical factors causing irritation and strain of the periosteal and other soft tissues attached to the medial posterior border of the tibia, which can cause shin pain and/or stress fractures. Radiographs should be taken to rule out bone and joint injury.

If there is a concomitant accessory soleus muscle present, which takes up space in the superficial posterior compartment, this may cause CECS. Sometimes, there is an accessory peroneus quartus muscle, which takes up space in the lateral compartment. All preoperative patients with compartment syndrome should be sent for an MRI to see if there is any abnormal pathology including accessory muscles, tendon (look for partial tears) and muscle pathology, soft tissue masses, bone pathology, and so forth. Any increased muscle mass within a fascial compartment can lead to CECS during exercise and the surgeon will need to debulk or excise the accessory muscles and perform the appropriate surgery along with the fasciotomy.

Other factors that must be excluded as a cause of leg pain are claudication and/or popliteal artery entrapment syndrome. With clinical suspicion, these patients should be sent for vascular testing, preferably functional testing, where the athlete runs and is immediately tested for signs of occlusion. This test may be compared with the baseline "at rest" vascular test.

The superficial peroneal nerve may be pinched (entrapped) as it exits through the lateral compartment leg fascia superficially. This may be detected by a positive provocation sign (direct finger compression elicits point tenderness) and/or confirmed by selective nerve block of 1 mL lidocaine, which should afford temporary relief of symptoms. The sural nerve also may get pinched as it exits the superficial posterior compartment fascia superficially in the distal one-third of the leg. Affected patients may complain of numbness/tingling to the lateral aspect of the foot or ankle. Check for a positive provocation sign directly over the sural nerve at the distal lateral leg. This nerve entrapment also should be verified by a selective nerve block. Nerve entrapment pain may be present at rest, with numbness or tingling along the path of the nerve and its branches, whereas the pain of CECS is usually severe during exercise activity.

Clinically, anterior and lateral CECS frequently occurs together and the superficial peroneal nerve found within the lateral compartment is the most common nerve to be affected by intracompartmental pressures. In those with longer histories of this condition, the patients may relate pains radiating to the dorsal lateral and dorsal aspect of the foot, which I have further diagnosed as intermediate dorsal cutaneous nerve and medial dorsal cutaneous nerve neuropraxia secondary to impingement of the superficial peroneal nerve. In those with chronic deep posterior exertional compartment syndrome, the saphenous nerve has been noted to demonstrate pain at the medial malleolus, and the anterior medial ankle, which extends to the medial big toe joint. So, if patients complain of distal symptoms and leg pains, especially during exercise, the practitioner should include "CECS-induced neuropraxia" in their differential diagnosis.

CHRONIC EXERTIONAL COMPARTMENT SYNDROME ETIOLOGY

My personal observations through clinical and surgical intervention of having tested and/or treated more than 100 patients with CECS are that some individuals are genetically predisposed to this syndrome due to their anatomic muscle composition. We have noted several patients who were twins, with both siblings experiencing this condition. Some individuals are born and exhibit high muscle tone and others develop hypertrophic muscles as a result of repeated exercise activities. This is very true for runners and dancers and anyone who performs repetitive activities. It is known that the lower extremity leg muscle volume may expand 20% during exercise from both increased capillary blood flow and the retaining of extracellular fluid (Puranen[5]). Ultimately, this intracompartment expansion increases the pressure within the enclosed fascia compartment. I personally believe that there is a similarity between CECS of the leg and that which is similar to tarsal tunnel syndrome. In the latter, there is an impingement of the posterior tibial nerve, often times by a surrounding hypertrophic muscle underneath the laciniate ligament. A common example of this is the presence of a hypertrophied flexor hallucis longus muscle in dancers and runners. Typically the flexor hallucis longus should be a tendon by the time it courses under the laciniate ligament, but I have often noted the presence of an enlarged or low lying flexor hallucis longus muscle under the laciniate ligament in patients with tarsal tunnel syndrome. If the athlete with tarsal tunnel syndrome persists in playing the sport with the pain, the muscle under the laciniate ligament may engorge with blood or extracellular fluid and he or she may develop a nerve impingement and resultant symptomatic burning, numbness, or muscle weakness to the plantar foot. Anything that increases pressure in the tarsal tunnel causes strain on the overlying laciniate ligament and impingement on the nerve. This also includes one with an inherently tight laciniate ligament. In CECS of the leg, there are similar findings in addition to intense pain and tightness.

Biomechanically speaking, I have not had great success nor has the literature supported treating patients with CECS by orthotic therapy. However, when there are biomechanical abnormalities, orthotics should be fabricated before considering surgical intervention. Detmer and colleagues[4] reported that 15% of their patients considered orthotics somewhat helpful, although it is unknown if the use of orthotics resolved their problems.

It has been my experience that some patients present with a small fascial herniation in the lower leg muscles, which may be indicative of CECS. If warranted by intracompartmental testing, appropriate completion of the fasciotomy should be performed.

As one's muscles develop through repetitive activities, it appears that the fascial coverings may not expand enough, grow, or accommodate for the increased muscle mass. On the other hand, the symptomatic patient with CECS may simply have been born with tight fascia that only becomes symptomatic during repetitive activities.

CECS occurs as a result of various factors, but always increases the intracompartmental pressures with resultant symptoms as discussed.

ANATOMY AND CLINICAL EXAMINATION

There are 4 muscle compartments in the lower extremities surrounded by fascia that are commonly tested in compartment syndrome. Detmer and colleagues[4] identified additional subcompartments in the legs, but most surgeons focus on the 4 compartments. Beyond the scope of this article, it should be known that there is also CECS of the foot that is documented in the peer-reviewed literature. The leg compartments include the anterior compartment, which consists of the anterior tibial, extensor hallucis longus, extensor digitorum longus, and peroneus tertius muscles. The lateral compartment consists of the peroneus longus and peroneus brevis muscles. The deep posterior compartment includes the posterior tibial, flexor digitorum longus, and the flexor hallucis longus muscles. The superficial posterior compartment includes the soleus, gastrocnemius, and plantaris muscles.

A key point to note is that the most consistent resolution of CECS leg pain/symptoms is rest, although athletes may be able to sit on the bench or stop running for 15 minutes or so and then return to activity, albeit for short periods of time and often at subpar levels. Most patients have no pain on palpation during their initial examination; however, if they were to run until they have their symptoms, they may have pain on palpation or they would be able to better identify the location of pain. After exhibiting their symptoms, patients should be asked to point their finger to the exact area(s) of their pain so that the clinician may better understand the area of potential fascial release.

TESTING FOR EXERTIONAL COMPARTMENT SYNDROME

The most reliable methods of quantifying exertional compartment syndrome is by taking intramuscular compartment pressures using the Stryker Intra-Compartmental Pressure Monitor System (Stryker, Kalamazoo, MI) by way of pressure testing as described by Whitesides and colleagues[6] and since simplified with use of the Stryker Quick Pressure Monitor Set, including diaphragm chamber and side-ported needle system (**Figs. 1** and **2**).

I typically test one leg in the athlete to spare the patient the discomfort of testing both legs. Although, if the test results are questionable, I will then test the opposite

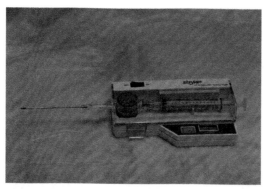

Fig. 1. Stryker intracompartmental monitor system. (*Courtesy of* Stryker, Kalamazoo, MI; with permission.)

leg if symptomatic. The athlete is placed supine on the examination table with his or her knee bent, so the sole of the foot is flat on the table. By having the lower leg upright, there is easy access to all the compartments. An indelible marker is used to circle the area for injection over each of the 4 compartments. The leg is then prepped with povidone-iodine solution. I raise a skin wheal within each circled area for each of the 4 compartments using 0.5 mL of 2% lidocaine plain. This helps reduce the superficial (skin stick) pain of the larger 18-gauge side-port needle. It is important not to anesthetize deep to the skin.

For the anterior compartment, the injection site is between the upper one-third and middle one-third of the anterior leg staying lateral to the tibia and directly over the anterior tibial muscle.

Be sure to zero balance the pressure monitor system holding the unit perpendicular to the leg and parallel to the examination table. Insert the side-port needle into the anterior tibial muscle (**Fig. 3**) approximately 1.5 to 2.0 cm deep and inject approximately 0.3 mL to 0.5 mL saline from the syringe into the muscle belly. Then record the pressure off the monitor once you reach an equilibrium state, which occurs when the LCD readout stops or fluctuates back and forth a few degrees mm Hg.

Repeat the procedure for the lateral compartment (**Fig. 4**), which should be lateral to the anterior compartment and over the area of the fibular shaft. Here, you are inserting

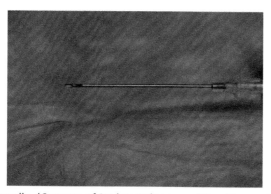

Fig. 2. Side-port needle. (*Courtesy of* Stryker, Kalamazoo, MI; with permission.)

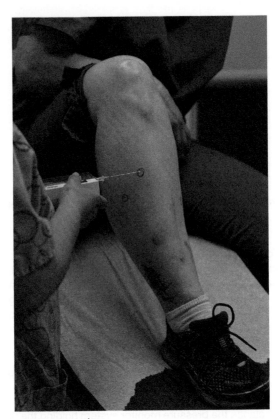

Fig. 3. Anterior compartment testing.

the needle perpendicular into the peroneus longus muscle belly in similar fashion as previously described. After the saline injection, record the pressure.

For the deep posterior compartment (**Fig. 5**), place the needle midway up the leg staying just posterior to the medial surface of the tibia, thereby staying anterior and avoiding the saphenous vein and nerve. The needle is inserted approximately 2.0 to 2.5 cm deep into the posterior tibial muscle belly and after the injection of 0.3 mL to 0.5 mL sterile saline, the pressure is recorded.

To measure the superficial posterior compartment (**Fig. 6**), which is more proximal up the leg, insert the needle into the medial head of the gastrocnemius. If the lateral head is more symptomatic, you should measure this pressure as well. Again, in a similar saline injection technique, measure the pressures.

The anterior and the lateral compartments are the most commonly involved compartments in CECS and when performing fasciotomies the anterior and lateral compartments are typically performed together. When the deep posterior or superficial compartments are involved, both compartments receive fasciotomies.

Plastic strip bandages are applied to cover each injection site. After recording the baseline pressures, have the patient run either on a treadmill or outside until the symptoms are reproduced. I have not found that cycling reproduces their symptoms as well as running. Once the athlete returns with the symptoms, the testing is repeated within 1 minute of cessation of activities. The plastic strip bandages are quickly removed and testing is repeated. The second round of injections is slightly less painful than the first

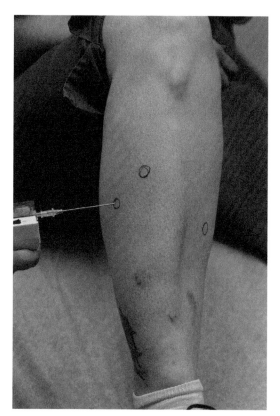

Fig. 4. Lateral compartment testing.

because the needle tract within the skin has already been established. Retest all the compartments in the same order as before and record all pressures.

A timer is used to wait 5 minutes and then all 4 compartments are once again injected with the saline and the pressures again recorded in the same order as previously.

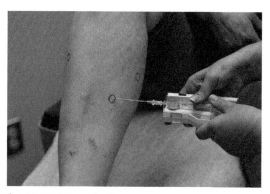

Fig. 5. Deep posterior compartment testing.

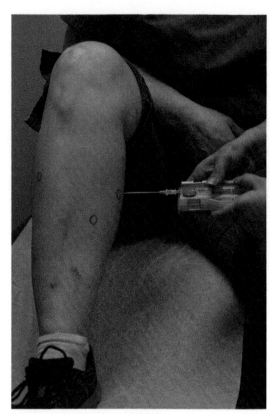

Fig. 6. Superficial posterior compartment testing.

Normal baseline pressures before exercise should be approximately 15 to 20 mm Hg. If the pressures are higher than this amount in the preexercise recordings, then exertional compartment syndrome has been established. If the immediate postexercise pressures increase greater than 30 mm Hg, then this is also considered pathologic. Finally, if the 5-minute postexercise measurements do not return to under 20 mm Hg, then this is also indicative of CECS. At any point of the 3 phases of testing where the pressures are increased higher than normal, then additional testing is not needed, but completing the test with multiple high-pressure recordings is more convincing.

There has been some recent CECS testing performed with functional MRI scanning followed by stress computed tomography (CT) angiography. The premise is that CECS may be caused by functional venous outflow obstruction. Treatment via CT and ultrasound-guided injection of botulinum toxin into the muscle adjacent to the area of venous compression has empirically been shown to help weaken a muscle or decrease spasm for several months and thereby reduce compression pressure on the obstructed vessel.[7]

PERFORMING THE CORRECTIVE FASCIOTOMY FOR CHRONIC EXERTIONAL COMPARTMENT SYNDROME

Once you have established the CECS diagnosis and conservative care measures have failed, you should proceed to the corrective fasciotomy. For a certain period of time, I performed the fasciotomies with a small incision, endoscopically assisted. However, I was not able to fully release the deep posterior compartment and identify unexpected accompanying pathology that could better be identified in the modified open technique herein discussed.

Apply a well-padded thigh tourniquet, but it is not necessary to inflate it unless an abnormal bleeder is present during surgery. General laryngeal mask airway (LMA) or other anesthesia is obtained. Either a popliteal nerve block is performed or one can block the common peroneal and saphenous nerves proximally. A sterile scrub, prep, and drape is always performed. I prefer to use the single incisional approach, which I have modified from that of Mubarak and Hargens.[2]

For the anterior and lateral compartments, make a linear longitudinal incision approximately 8 cm long, midway up the leg between the tibial crest and fibula shaft (**Fig. 7**). Sharply dissect the incision to the level of the subcutaneous tissues down to the layer of the overlying fascia. In addition, one should finger sweep dissect the subcutaneous tissues away from the fascia, so that an unobstructed cut of the fascia may be performed (**Fig. 8**). Right angle retractors such as Army-Navy or lighted breast retractors should be used to help visualize the fasciotomy. You should be able to identify the intermuscular septum separating the anterior and lateral compartments (**Fig. 9**). Meticulously dissect the septum with tenotomy or small Metzenbaum scissors, until you locate the superficial peroneal nerve, which may be found within the intermuscular septum (**Fig. 10**) or just lateral to the intermuscular septum within the lateral compartment. Occasionally, this nerve runs just anterior to the intermuscular septum within the anterior compartment. Inspect this nerve for any obvious signs of pathology, entrapment, or adhesions and free them if necessary.

The anterior compartment will lie anterior to the intermuscular septum. Make a nick with a scalpel blade into the overlying fascia. Using a 10-inch to 12-inch Metzenbaum straight scissor, cut the overlying anterior fascia proximally toward the patella tubercle and distally toward the anterior aspect of the lateral malleolus (see **Fig. 7**). This cut is made by using the sharp portion of the scissors distally, holding the scissors open 1 cm and sliding the scissors along the fascia to cut it much like a tape cutter is used to remove athletic tape.

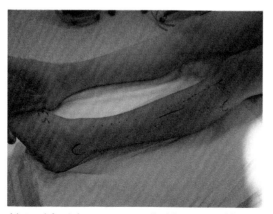

Fig. 7. Anterior and lateral fascial compartment incision. Dotted lines indicate fasciotomy: anterior compartment fascia is cut proximally toward patella tubercle and distally toward anterior aspect of lateral malleolus. Lateral compartment fascia is cut proximally toward fibular head and distally toward posterior aspect of lateral malleolus.

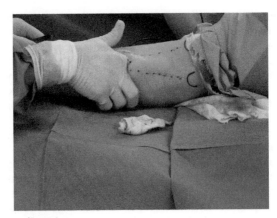

Fig. 8. Finger sweep dissection.

Release of the lateral compartment is performed after a nick is made in the fascia, lateral/posterior to the superficial peroneal nerve. The scissors are directed proximally toward the fibular head and distally toward the posterior aspect of the lateral malleolus (see **Fig. 7**). It is important to visualize and slide the tips of the scissors so that only the fascia is released and one stays posterior to the superficial peroneal nerve. By keeping the tips of the scissors along the fascia, one also avoids cutting the superficial branches of the peroneal nerve. While cutting the fascia, a slight upward pressure should be maintained to avoid cutting muscle tissue, which causes bleeding, and is also why blunt-tipped scissors are appropriate (**Figs. 11** and **12**).

To release the superficial posterior and deep posterior compartments, I recommend making one 8-cm-long linear longitudinal incision approximately 2 cm posterior to the palpated medial posterior margin of the tibia (**Fig. 13**). The incision is deepened to the level of the fascia. The subcutaneous and fatty tissues are separated from the overlying fascia using finger sweep dissection. At this time, one should be able to identify the saphenous nerve and vein, which is typically just posterior-medial to the tibia shaft overlying the deep posterior compartment. Check the saphenous nerve for overlying adhesions and free them if necessary. Retract the saphenous nerve and vein anteriorly

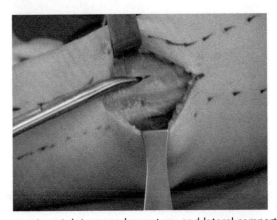

Fig. 9. Anterior compartment, intermuscular septum, and lateral compartment.

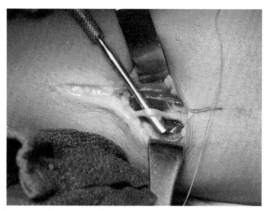

Fig. 10. Superficial peroneal nerve within the intermuscular septum.

and carefully make a superficial transverse incision and, using tenotomy or small Metzenbaum scissors, identify the intermuscular septum between the deep posterior and superficial posterior compartments.

The superficial posterior compartment fasciotomy is then performed by making a nick into the fascia over the medial portion of the soleus muscle (mid leg) and then directing the scissors proximally and diagonally across or along the medial head of the gastrocnemius staying posterior to the intermuscular septum (see **Fig. 13**). You should free the superficial posterior fascia as far distal as the musculotendinous junction. Additional release of fascia may be performed to the lateral gastrocnemius head if needed, being careful to avoid the deeper sural nerve.

To release the fascia encasing the deep posterior compartment, make a nick in the fascia, and slide the scissors proximally in a linear longitudinal manner aiming the scissor tips proximally, straight upward toward the tibial crest staying anterior to the intermuscular septum and then distally downward staying posterior to the medial malleolus (see **Fig. 13**). Be sure to retract the saphenous nerve and vein anteriorly during the proximal cut. While releasing the deep posterior compartment, it may be necessary to release the "soleus bridge," which is a connection of the soleus muscle via soft tissue to the

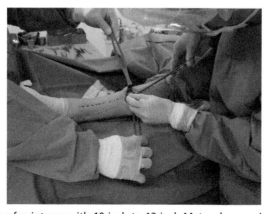

Fig. 11. Performing fasciotomy with 10-inch to 12-inch Metzenbaum scissor.

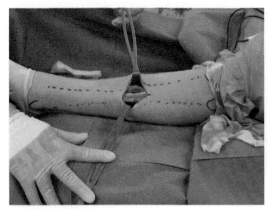

Fig. 12. Completed anterior and lateral fasciotomy.

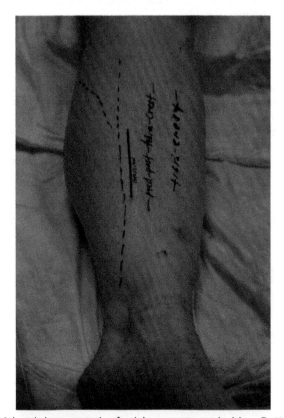

Fig. 13. Superficial and deep posterior fascial compartment incision. Dotted lines indicate fasciotomy: superficial posterior compartment fascia is cut proximally diagonally across or along the medial head of the gastrocnemius. Deep posterior compartment fascia is cut proximally toward the tibial crest and distally toward the posterior aspect of the medial malleolus.

periosteum of the mid tibia. This should be performed bluntly with a finger sweep motion or with the use of a blunt elevator to free the area between the soleus and the tibia.

If there is concomitant chronic shin splint pain, then one should palpate the periosteal tissues along the tibia where complaints of pains have been identified. If there are any areas of fibrosis or scarification noted, this area of periosteal tissue may be excised.[8] During surgery, I have often noted micro-nodules along the medial distal tibia border. After excising the nodules or stripping a small amount of periosteal tissue, I rasp the area to smooth any sharp or irritating border of the tibia. I believe that rasping the bone also promotes regrowth or adherence of sharpey's fibers or periosteal tissue to the overlying soft tissues.

Additionally, if there is any concomitant gastrocnemius equinus deformity then the medial gastrocnemius aponeurosis is cut in a transverse manner from medial to lateral just distal to the gastrocnemius muscle (make sure to see the soleus muscle deep to it) until the appropriate ankle dorsiflexion is achieved. Usually no more than 2.5 cm is transected medially to avoid exorbitant weakening of calf plantar flexion.

The surgical sites are then irrigated with sterile saline solution. The fascia is not sutured. It is my preference to insert a closed suction drain for 24 to 48 hours for the posterior compartment and another for the anterior/lateral compartments to help reduce the incidence of hematoma. The subcutaneous tissues are closed in standard technique with absorbable suture. Staples are often used for the skin. The surgical site is dressed with sterile gauze and elastic bandages. The patient is placed in a removable below-knee walker-type cast or well-padded posterior splint cast.

POSTOPERATIVE CARE

The patient follows up within 24 to 48 hours for removal of the closed suctioned drain. Patients are then instructed on range-of-motion exercises to be performed within a few days of surgery, several times per day. This includes toe flexion and extension exercises, ankle range of motion exercises, and knee flexion and extension exercises. Patients remain in a walker-type boot cast non–weight bearing for 3 weeks. Suture and/or skin staples are removed at approximately 3 weeks and then patients attend rehabilitation. Patients may perform upper body exercises and/or cycling soon after the surgery, but must elevate their legs afterward to compensate for any swelling.

POSTOPERATIVE COMPLICATIONS

In my experience the most common complication has been hematoma formation. This may be evident from dissecting through small vessels or due to inadvertent cutting of muscle tissue while performing the procedure(s). A surgeon can either perform the procedures wet and cauterize any bleeders as encountered, or use a tourniquet and let it down before closure to check for bleeders. Hematoma (and seroma) formation delays the healing process and has a higher incidence of infection. One must be aggressive with physical therapy when a hematoma or seroma is identified and apply heat packs, massage, and electrical muscle stimulation to assist in breaking up the hematoma. If necessary, aspirations should be performed to diagnose either hematoma or seroma and to relieve pressure and allow for better soft tissue healing. To be on the safe side, I have been using a closed suction drain in all recent cases and have not had any more issues with hematoma formation.

Wound dehiscence is another complication, especially when performing additional surgery for chronic shin splints that requires dissection along the posterior-medial tibia. Wound dehiscence can delay surgical healing, leave a hypertrophic or unsightly scar, and expose the soft tissue to infection. It is usually caused by significant swelling with tension on the skin or improper closure of the skin. If the wound margins gap open, then it is important to bring the patient back to the operating room and undermine the skin. Release the tension and then apply either retention sutures or an external tissue expander device. This is usually augmented with new sutures applied after a few days and the retention sutures or tissue expander removed.

During surgery, patients are usually placed on intraoperative intravenous antibiotics, and after surgery they continue with prophylactic oral antibiotics, so infection has been rare. Localized skin hypoesthesia is often a complication. This is a fairly common complication after any leg surgery. It is possible that during the procedure, the surgeon may cut a small aberrant nerve branch or small nerve(s) within the skin incision site are sacrificed. As with any surgical procedure, potential risks and complications must be discussed and documented with the patient before the surgery.

In summary, increased tissue pressure within a fascial compartment may be the result of any increase in volume within its contents or any decrease in size of the fascial covering or due to any distensibility of the fascial covering (eg, patients with thickened fascia). Therefore, the initial clinical diagnosis of CECS is made by a careful history and by exclusion of other maladies and confirmed by compartmental syndrome testing. Once the practitioner makes the proper diagnoses of CECS, through clinical examination and intracompartmental testing, surgical fasciotomy along with ancillary procedures should allow the athlete to return to competitive activity.

REFERENCES

1. Mavor GE. The anterior tibial syndrome. J Bone Joint Surg Br 1956;38-B(2):513–7.
2. Mubarak SJ, Hargens AR. Acute compartment syndromes. Surg Clin North Am 1983;63(3):539–65.
3. Amendola A, Rorabeck CH, Vellett D, et al. The use of magnetic resonance imaging in exertional compartment syndromes. Am J Sports Med 1990;18(1): 29–34.
4. Detmer DE, Sharpe K, Sufit RL, et al. Chronic compartment syndrome: diagnoses, management, and outcomes. Am J Sports Med 1985;13(3):162–70.
5. Puranen J. The medial tibial syndrome: exercise ischaemia in the medial fascial compartment of the leg. J Bone Joint Surg Br 1974;56-B(4):712–5.
6. Whitesides TE, Haney TC, Harada H, et al. A simple method for tissue pressure determination. Arch Surg 1975;110:1311–3.
7. McGinley JC. Lecture presentation. Denver (CO): Association of Extremity Nerve Surgeons; 2015.
8. Yates B, Allen MJ, Barnes MR. Outcome of surgical treatment of medial tibial stress syndrome. J Bone Joint Surg Am 2003;85-A(10):1974–80.

FURTHER READINGS

Braver RT. How to test and treat exertional compartment syndrome. Podiatry Today 2002.
Jarvinnen M, Aho H, Niittymaki S. Results of the surgical treatment of the medial tibial syndrome in athletes. Int J Sports Med 1989;10(1):55–7.
Lutz LJ, Goodenough GK, Detmer DE. Chronic compartment syndrome. Am Fam Physician 1989;39(2):191–6.
Matsen FA. Compartmental syndrome clinics orthopaedics and related research. No. 113, Nov-Dec 1975.
Michael RH, Holder LER. The soleus syndrome—a cause of medial tibial stress. Am J Sports Med 1985;13(2):87–94.

Pedowitz RA, Hargens AR, Mubarak SJ, et al. Modified criteria for the objective diagnosis of chronic compartment syndrome of the leg. Am J Sports Med 1990;18(1):35–40.

Peterson DA, Stinson W, Carter J. Bilateral accessory soleus: a report on four patients with partial fasciectomy. Foot Ankle 1993;14(5):284–8.

Rettig AC, McCarroll JR, Hahn RG. Chronic compartment syndrome- surgical intervention in 12 cases. Phys Sportsmed 1991;19(4):63–70.

Stryker surgical: intra-compartmental pressure moniter system maintenance manual and operating instructions. 295-1-72. 10/89.

Turnipseed W, Detmer DE, Girdley F. Chronic compartment syndrome. Ann Surg 1989;210(4):557–62.

Veith RG, Matsen FA, Newell SG. Recurrent anterior compartmental syndromes. Phys Sportsmed 1980;8(11):80–8.

Wiley JP, Clement DB, Doyle DL, et al. A primary care perspective of chronic compartment syndrome of the leg. Phys Sportsmed 1987;15(3):111–20.

Zammit J, Singh D. The peroneus quartus muscle. J Bone Joint Surg Br 2003;85-B(8):1134–7.

Management of Painful Recurrent Intermetatarsal Neuroma Using Processed Porcine Extracellular Matrix Material

CrossMark

A Case Report

Robert G. Parker, DPM[a], Orlando Merced-O'Neil, BS, RN, CTBS[b],*

KEYWORDS

- Nerve wrap • Recurrent neuroma • Stump neuroma
- Intermetatarsal stump neuroma • True neuroma
- Processed porcine extracellular matrix nerve wrap

KEY POINTS

- Painful recurrent stump neuromas are common following transection of a nerve after initial interdigital neuroma excision or even excision of a stump neuroma.
- After excising a stump neuroma, processed porcine extracellular matrix is a good material to cap the proximal nerve as a deterrent for recurrent neuroma formation.
- This article discusses capping material characteristics and considers factors that may contribute to clinical success for treating recurrent stump neuromas.

INTRODUCTION

Several large studies indicate that the failure rate for the first-time excision of interme-tatarsal neuroma ranges from 10% to 15%, with 1 study showing as high as nearly 50%[1] with recurrent stump neuroma as the most common complication.[2,3] Forefoot neuromas such as Morton and Hauser (second intermetatarsal) are the only nerve en-trapments that are routinely excised, and it is done less often in Joplin (first medial plantar hallucal) and Iselin (lateral plantar digital) nerves. This article lists all the forefoot plantar entrapments because there is a tendency, in general medicine, to call all fore-foot entrapments in this area Morton entrapments.[4] A recurrent stump neuroma can cause significant pain to the patient, as well as physical impairment, psychological

[a] American Board of Foot and Ankle Surgery, Houston, TX, USA; [b] AxoGen, Inc, Alachua, FL, USA
* Corresponding author. 400 Saddle Horn Drive, Bandera, TX 78003.
E-mail address: omerced-oneill@axogeninc.com

Clin Podiatr Med Surg 33 (2016) 235–242
http://dx.doi.org/10.1016/j.cpm.2015.11.001
0891-8422/16/$ – see front matter © 2016 Elsevier Inc. All rights reserved.

distress, and frustration for both patient and surgeon. Stump neuromas are a naturally occurring event after a nerve has been transected as the proximal nerve segment attempts to restore continuity. The proximal nerve forms multiple regenerating axons in various directions and without direction a bulb-shaped tangle of nerve and scar forms. Only destruction of the nerve cell body inhibits axonal regeneration completely and currently there is no procedure that is consistently successful in preventing stump or end-bulb neuroma formation.

In the event of painful recurrent intermetatarsal stump neuroma that does not respond to conservative treatment, surgical intervention is needed and additional measures, outside of simple resection, are often used to prevent further recurrence. A variety of surgical treatments has been explored in order to prevent end-stump neuroma formation; however, there is no panacea or any universally accepted gold standard of treatment. On surgical removal of end-stump neuromas, it is desirable to limit the axonal outgrowth into surrounding tissue, minimize scar tissue around the nerve, and reduce stress on the nerve by redirecting it to an area of reduced pressure and friction. Covering the nerve stump mechanically isolates it from the inflammatory environment and prevents interaction with surrounding neurotrophic factors produced as a result of nerve trauma. The most widely used methods of nerve covering may be capping the nerve stump or burying it in a suitable nearby anatomic structure such as muscle, or a combination of both. Various capping materials, including autologous tissue, synthetic material, and xenograft, have been introduced as a treatment modality; however, the results have been inconsistent and the material options leave something to be desired. Autologous tissues have shown favorable results but there are limitations associated with harvesting and availability. Identification of an alternative cap material that provides similar benefits to autologous tissue and is also readily available and technically simple to use is desired.

This article presents the novel use of processed porcine extracellular matrix (ECM) material to cap the proximal stump after removal of a recurrent intermetatarsal neuroma of the second intermetatarsal space. The technique uses a 2-fold isolation strategy in which the proximal end of the resected nerve is capped and then translocated into intrinsic muscle. Characteristics of the novel nerve cap material combined with surgical technique may contribute to the patient's clinical improvement and are discussed in this report.

CASE REPORT

The patient was a 49-year-old woman who presented with numbness, burning sensation, and sharp pain in the forefoot area at the base of the second and third toes. It is also typical to have a tethering or pulling on dorsiflexion of the foot where the stump neuroma is scarred and adhering to tissue such as the skin and the fascia. About 9 months before her initial examination, the patient underwent surgery at an outside institution to remove a Hauser neuroma in the second intermetatarsal area of the right foot. After surgery, the patient developed more pain than before the initial surgery, as well as the sensation of walking on pebbles. She had multiple injections postoperatively without any effect and was referred to the author's institution. Deep tendon reflexes, vibratory sensation, and Wartenberg pinwheel sensations were within normal limits in all anatomic areas with the exception of the triangular area at the base of the second and third toes and forefoot where the symptoms of pain were manifested. Examination revealed that the second interspace was tender to dorsal-plantar compression compared with the other interspaces, which were pain free. Based on the physical examination, a true neuroma or stump neuroma of the second interspace was diagnosed with entrapment of the stump tethered in an apparent ball of scar.

The patient was taken to the operating room approximately 19 months from the initial surgical removal of the Hauser neuroma. From a plantar approach, a 5-cm longitudinal incision was made over the suspected site of the neuroma, between the metatarsal heads of the interspace. The incision was carried deep using sharp and blunt dissection until scar tissue and nerve were identified (**Fig. 1**). A mass of scar tissue and tethered end-bulb neuroma was visualized. Attention was turned to neurolysis of the second intermetatarsal branch of the medial plantar nerve from the virgin proximal aspect of the nerve branches to the distal end-bulb or stump neuroma area. The neuroma was completely freed from the tissue bed (**Fig. 2**). Once freed, the stump neuroma was resected distally. The proximal end of the end-bulb neuroma was resected until healthy nerve tissue was visualized, noted by punctate interfascicular bleeding and nerve tissue that was soft to palpation (**Fig. 3**). The stump neuroma was then sent to pathology.

The fresh terminal nerve ending was wrapped using AxoGuard Nerve Protector (AxoGen Inc, Alachua, FL), a processed porcine ECM wrap. A wrap length of 20 mm was selected to fit the nerve stump diameter without compression of the fascicles. The wrap was secured to itself using 3 GEM Titanium Hemostatic MicroClips (Synovis, Birmingham, AL) (**Fig. 4**). The open end of the protective wrap was folded on itself and was sealed using another MicroClip so as to prevent axonal escape (**Fig. 5**). The nerve and wrap complex was then translocated and implanted into the intrinsic muscle belly. Note that neurolysis or simple decompression of nerves should never be splinted because neurogliding, or travel of nerves in the opened tunnels, helps to minimize scarring into surrounding tissue. When the fresh proximal end of a nerve is translocated, it must have slack at the most extended position of the foot to prevent pull-out of the implanted nerve. Splinting is an option here if the surgeon chooses. On completion of the procedure, hemostasis was achieved and the incision was irrigated and closed. A sterile compressive dressing was first applied, followed by application of a well-padded posterior splint in order to keep the foot in a position of neutral dorsiflexion.

Removal of the stump neuroma, capping of the fresh nerve ending with ECM wrap material, and burial of the fresh nerve ending in the muscle bed provided excellent pain relief.

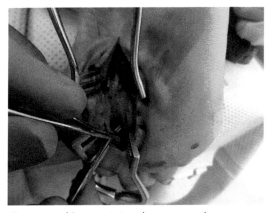

Fig. 1. Initial dissection, second intermetatarsal space scar tissue.

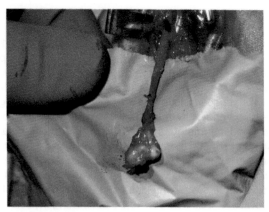

Fig. 2. Stump or true neuroma isolated.

DISCUSSION

Frequently resulting after the transection of a nerve, terminal stump neuromas may cause debilitating pain and functional impairment. When conservative treatments fail, surgical options are needed to remove the recurrent neuroma, prevent future axonal outgrowth, and isolate the nerve in a low-impact, tensionless environment. Burying of the proximal normal nerve, once the end-bulb or stump neuroma has been excised, into a nearby anatomic structure has been investigated as a means to isolate the stump from surrounding tissues and nerve growth factors. Several techniques have been documented, including burying in muscle, vein, and bone.[5–8] Wolfort and Dellon[7] reported clinical success implanting the interdigital nerve stump into the intrinsic muscle in the midarch of the foot, which was selected because it has little excursion and does not place tension on the nerve stump. All 13 patients with 17 nerve resections reported good or excellent relief of interdigital pain symptoms and no complications were reported. Although promising, experimental studies have indicated that neuroma may still form within the muscle. I have personally revised 2 cases referred to me even after the nerve was translocated and implanted into muscle. It is a different type that contains less connective tissue and is formed mainly by sensory

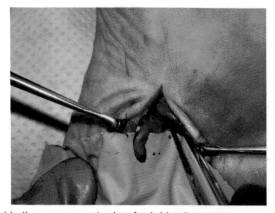

Fig. 3. Stump/end-bulb neuroma excised to fresh bleeding nerve.

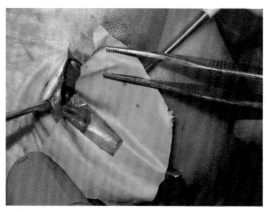

Fig. 4. Initial wrap of AxoGuard Nerve Protector secured proximally with GEM titanium MicroClips.

neurons. Although typically smaller, these neuromas have been reported to be painful in certain circumstances.[9] One of the 2 I experienced was without burning and tingling, but with debilitating cramping in the arch.

Capping of a nerve after excision of the stump neuroma has also been well documented in the literature as an effective and widely used method of preventing neuroma formation. The nerve cap provides a physical barrier to isolate the nerve from surrounding inflammation and scar tissue while also serving to block surrounding growth factors,

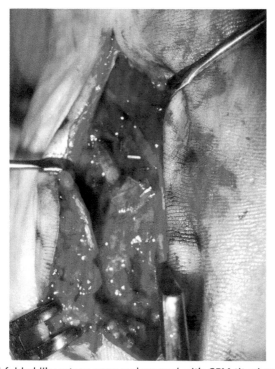

Fig. 5. Open end folded like a taco wrap and secured with GEM titanium MicroClips.

thereby attenuating the regenerative response.[2,8,10,11] Various capping materials have been used in an attempt to treat recurrent stump neuromas, but an optimal material has yet to be identified.

Epineural capping techniques have been widely reported in the literature. Sunderland[12] showed that normal epineurium prevents the lateral outgrowth of regenerating axons and concluded that intact epineurium can control terminal neuroma formation by isolating neural tissues from surrounding connective tissues. Several different mechanisms of epineural caps have been proposed but the consistent problem of axonal escape remains.[13] Yuksel and colleagues[13] used 3 variations on epineural barriers with limited success. They attribute the poor outcomes to microsurgical suturing, stating that it does not provide a tight enough seal to prevent axonal sprouts from escaping. Other methods, such as laser sealing or gluing of epineurium, have been explored, but with disappointing results.[14]

Biological tissues offer an appealing barrier material because of their tendency to remodel, which is thought to improve local vascularity.[15] Covering of nerve stumps using free vascularized tissue, including fat and muscle, has been documented in the literature as having limited success.[15,16] These tissues are often bulky and require complex procedures with potential donor morbidity.[17] Several studies have documented the use of free vein caps on terminal stumps.[10] Veins, like other autologous tissues, provide a material that can be remodeled, bringing vascularity to the nerve, and are available throughout the body. Despite these beneficial features, vein caps are imperfect because they require sacrifice of surrounding vein, and can be surgically complex, time-consuming procedures. In addition, surgeons have faced technical issues using vein because veins typically present a diameter discrepancy between the vein lumen and the nerve and have a tendency to collapse.[17]

Off-the-shelf products provide readily available cap material without the need for autologous harvest and the potential for donor site morbidity. These options allow nerve diameter matching and are less surgically intensive procedures. Several studies have documented the use of silicon devices in the treatment of terminal stump neuromas.[18] Swanson and colleagues[18] described the effects of cap size on the nerve stump. They found that excessive length of a cap leads to ischemic necrosis of the distal tip of the nerve and observed neuroma formation when caps were much larger in diameter than the nerve stump. As a result, they suggested a cap length/diameter ratio of 5:1 and applied this concept in a clinical setting with good results. One patient reported continued discomfort of the silicon-capped nerve and required revision surgery. Although silicon provides a permanent nonresorbable barrier, it is a rigid, bulky material that encapsulates and may restrict the nerve as it moves. This restriction can lead to fibrosis where the nerve enters the conduits as well as chronic nerve compression requiring removal of the device.[17,18]

More recently, type I bovine collagen tubes have been used as capping material in lower extremities with considerable success. Gould and colleagues[17] reported a success rate of 85% when recurrent neuromas were removed, capped with collagen tubes, and redirected to a low-impact area of the foot. Of 69 nerve conduit constructs, 30 were painless at final outcome (43%). Ten nerves (15%) in 7 patients had unsatisfactory outcomes, classified as severe pain as bad as or worse than before surgery. Surgical revision of failed intermetatarsal capping was required in 2 nerves. Gould and colleagues[17] suggested that tightness at the entrance or within the conduit or kinking of the conduit could be factors. Type I bovine collagen material is eventually broken down and resorbed by the body and has been shown to elicit inflammatory responses caused by breakdown products. In addition, the collagen tube does not provide a permanent barrier to contain regenerating axons, which have been shown to grow years after transection.

The variable results and technical obstacles of materials reported in the literature led the author to seek an alternative material option. Acellular ECM material derived from porcine small intestinal submucosa was chosen as the capping material in this case because it has many of the desirable properties of autologous tissue but is technically simpler to work with and eliminates the time and morbidity associated with autograft harvest.[19] In a rabbit sciatic nerve model, the material was shown to quickly vascularize in situ and remodel into a connective tissue structure similar to nerve epineurium. As previously mentioned, nerve epineurium covering a nerve stump prevents lateral outgrowth of nerve fibers.[12] The ability of the material to revascularize may be beneficial to the nerve stump by bringing blood supply to the injury site and facilitating wound healing.[19] In contrast, materials that do not revascularize, such as silicone, have been reported to lead to ischemic necrosis of the nerve stump.[18] The wrap is readily available in a variety of sizes to allow for proper stump diameter matching, which is another important consideration in preventing neuroma formation.[18] Unlike other off-the-shelf options, processed porcine ECM has a low profile and has the flexibility to conform to the nerve without constricting it.

A 2-fold isolation approach was used in this case with the ECM cap in place to prevent axonal outgrowth into the surrounding tissues and the nerve-cap complex implanted in the low-impact protective intrinsic muscle of the foot. The positive clinical outcome from this case suggests that processed porcine ECM is a promising nerve cap material option to address these difficult recurrent stump neuroma cases. An understanding of the natural response to axotomy combined with the clinical evidence involving the mechanism of nerve caps and isolation of the nerve stump within the muscle offers a reasonable explanation for the success of this case.

ACKNOWLEDGMENTS

Erick DeVinney, Vice President of Clinical and Translational Sciences, AxoGen Inc, for information and technical education on the molecular and scientific aspects of AxoGuard Nerve Protector ECM.

REFERENCES

1. Richardson DR, Murphy GA, Womack JW. Long-term evaluation of interdigital neuroma treated by surgical excision. Foot Ankle Int 2008;29(6):574–7.
2. Wu K. Morton's interdigital neuroma: a clinical review of its etiology, treatment, and results. J Foot Ankle Surg 1996;35(2):112–9.
3. Malay DS. Recurrent intermetatarsal neuroma. In: McGlamry ED, editor. Reconstructive surgery of the foot and leg. Tucker (GA): Podiatry Institute; 1989. p. 321–4. Update 89.
4. Jarvis J, Barrett SL. Equinus deformity as a factor in forefoot nerve entrapment: treatment with endoscopic gastrocnemius recession. J Am Podiatr Med Assoc 2005;95(5):464–8.
5. Mobbs RJ, Vonau M, Blum P. Treatment of painful peripheral neuroma by vein implantation. J Clin Neurosci 2003;10(3):338–9.
6. Mass DP, Ciano MC, Tortosa R, et al. Treatment of painful hand neuromas by their transfer into bone. Plast Reconstr Surg 1984;74:182–5.
7. Wolfort S, Dellon L. Treatment of recurrent neuroma of the interdigital nerve by implantation of the proximal nerve into muscle in the arch of the foot. J Foot Ankle Surg 2001;40(6):404–10.

8. Koch H, Haas F, Hubmer M. Treatment of painful neuroma by resection and nerve stump transplantation into a vein. Ann Plast Surg 2003;51(1):45–50.

9. Otfinowski J, Pawelec A, Kaluza J. Implantation of peripheral neural stump into muscle and its effect on the development of posttraumatic neuroma. Pol J Pathol 1994;45:195–202.

10. Galeano M, Manasseri B, Risitano G, et al. A free vein graft cap influences neuroma formation after nerve transection. Microsurgery 2009;29:568–72.

11. Kakinoki R, Ikeguchi R, Matsumoto T, et al. Treatment of painful peripheral neuromas by vein implantation. Int Orthop 2003;27:60–4.

12. Sunderland S. The connective tissues of peripheral nerves. Brain 1965;88:841–54.

13. Yuksel F, Kislaoglu E, Durak N, et al. Prevention of painful neuromas by epineural ligatures, flaps, and grafts. Br J Plast Surg 1997;50:182–5.

14. Rahimi C, Muehleman F. Epineurial capping via Surgitron and the reduction of stump neuromas in the rat. J Foot Surg 1992;31(2):124–8.

15. Vaienti L, Merle M, Villani F, et al. Fat grafting according to Coleman for the treatment of radial nerve neuromas. Plast Reconstr Surg 2010;126:676–8.

16. Thomas M, Stirrat A, Birch R, et al. Freeze-thawed muscle grafting for painful cutaneous neuromas. J Bone Joint Surg Br 1994;76B(3):474–6.

17. Gould J, Naranje S, McGwin G, et al. Use of collagen conduits in management of painful neuromas of the foot and ankle. Foot Ankle Int 2013;34:932–40.

18. Swanson A, Boeve N, Lumsden R. The prevention and treatment of amputation neuromata by silicon capping. J Hand Surg 1977;2(1):70–8.

19. Kokkalis Z, Pu C, Small G, et al. Assessment of processed porcine extracellular matrix as a protective barrier in a rabbit nerve wrap model. J Reconstr Microsurg 2011;27:19–28.

Current Diagnosis and Treatment of Superficial Fibular Nerve Injuries and Entrapment

Peter J. Bregman, DPM[a],*, Mark Schuenke, PhD[b]

KEYWORDS

- Ankle • Epineurium • Leg • Nerve sheath • Neurolysis • Nerve repair • Neuroma

KEY POINTS

- Identification and treatment of entrapment of the SFN are important topics of discussion for foot and ankle surgeons, because overlooking the diagnosis can lead to permanent nerve damage.
- Some patients present with symptoms localized in their feet and, unless the examining clinician takes the time and makes the effort to look more proximal, the diagnosis may be missed if it is related to an SFN entrapment.
- Early diagnosis and treatment are crucial to avoidance of permanent nerve damage.
- Depending on the pathology, either decompression or, in cases of nerve trauma, neurectomy with implantation of the affected nerve into muscle with or without a nerve allograft is indicated. For this reason, peripheral nerve surgeons have to understand the rationale for and the technical maneuvers required to execute external neurolysis, nerve excision, and endoneurolysis, each of which is a fundamental element of basic peripheral nerve surgery.
- With the proper tools and skills, surgeons are able to help patients with symptomatic SFN entrapment, patients who often present in some degree of desperation, with the peripheral nerve surgeon as a last resort.

Financial Disclosures: None reported.

Conflict of Interest: Dr P.J. Bregman is a current member and past president of the Association of Extremity Nerve Surgeons. This is a nonprofit organization dedicated to the study of peripheral nerve disease and injuries to the lower extremity. The group is also involved in research and the teaching of peripheral nerve surgery.

[a] Bregman Peripheral Neuropathy Center of Las Vegas, Foot, Ankle, and Hand Center of Las Vegas, 7135 West Sahara Avenue Suite 201, Las Vegas, NV 89117, USA; [b] College of Osteopathic Medicine, University of New England, Biddeford, ME 04005, USA
* Corresponding address.
E-mail address: drbregman@gmail.com

Clin Podiatr Med Surg 33 (2016) 243–254
http://dx.doi.org/10.1016/j.cpm.2015.12.007
0891-8422/16/$ – see front matter © 2016 Elsevier Inc. All rights reserved.

Video content accompanies this article at http://www.podiatric.theclinics.com

Much has been written on the diagnosis and treatment of superficial peroneal nerve (SPN) entrapment. The SPN is now known as the superficial fibular nerve (SFN). This article uses the abbreviation SFN to represent both. This commentary attempts to provide insight into this often misdiagnosed and certainly underdiagnosed lower extremity pathology. Some tips and pearls also are presented to aid in the diagnosis and treatment of SFN entrapment or injury. Some patients present with symptoms localized in their feet and, unless an examining clinician takes the time and makes the effort to look more proximal, the diagnosis may be missed if it is related to an SFN entrapment.

Depending on the pathology, either decompression or, in cases of nerve trauma, neurectomy with implantation of the affected nerve into muscle with or without a nerve allograft is indicated. For this reason, peripheral nerve surgeons have to understand the rationale for and the technical maneuvers required to execute external neurolysis, nerve excision, and endoneurolysis, each of which is a fundamental element of basic peripheral nerve surgery. It is also important for surgeons to become skilled in the art of diagnostic blocks, to intimately know the anatomy of peripheral nerves in the lower extremity, and to identify and treat entrapment of the SFN (or any other named, anatomic nerve) inferior to the knee. With the proper tools and skills, surgeons are able to help patients with symptomatic SFN entrapment, patients who often present in some degree of desperation, with the peripheral nerve surgeon as a last resort.

To the authors' knowledge, Kernohan and colleagues,[1] in 1985, were the first to publish an article describing entrapment of the SFN, where they referred to Henry's 1945 publication, entitled "Extensile Approach." Styf,[2] in 1989, stated that the incidence of SFN entrapment causing anterior lateral leg pain was probably higher than suggested in the literature at that time. Donovan and colleagues[3] also stated that entrapment neuropathies of the knee, leg, ankle, and foot were often underdiagnosed, because clinical and electrodiagnostic evaluation was not always reliable. The nomenclature of the SPN has gradually become to be known as the SFN. This change in nomenclature was made by the anatomists and more or less has been adopted by most investigators.

A patient with peripheral nerve pathology can be treated surgically or nonsurgically, depending on the specific diagnosis, and appropriate surgical management may involve a neurectomy or a decompression of 1 or more nerves. There are a variety of conservative treatment options, of which nerve gliding or nerve flossing (another term for nerve gliding) is the most commonly used and most effective.[4] This involves specific maneuvers usually performed by a physical therapist that places a stretch on the entrapped nerve and also involves techniques to break up any adhesions of the surrounding fascia or scar tissue. The patient is given a specific home exercise program that incorporates these specific techniques. The concept of decompression of a peripheral nerve, and not those localized to the lower extremity, still seems controversial. The peer-reviewed literature pertaining to nerve entrapment of the upper extremity is voluminous. As the population becomes more obese and the diagnosis of diabetes mellitus more prevalent, symptomatic peripheral nerve conditions will concomitantly increase in frequency, and timely and accurate diagnosis and subsequent treatment of these peripheral nerve entrapments have become ever more important because a delay in treatment can lead to permanent nerve damage. Donovan and colleagues[3] stated that if the symptoms of nerve entrapment persist for 2 to 3 months, then surgical decompression is usually required to prevent permanent nerve damage. This statement accentuates the importance of early diagnosis and early intervention. This also reinforces the idea that clinicians using nonsurgical techniques should be careful so as to avoid prolonged efforts that are not showing adequate results, again because permanent damage to the nerve could be present. Clinicians should be monitoring the progress of any treatment whether it is surgical or nonsurgical. This is accomplished by using 2-point discrimination, pinprick test, Pressure Specified Sensory Device (PSSD), and electrodiagnostic testing. The subjective data from a patient, such as pain relief and restoration of sensation, are also a way to document improvement. Improvement in the Tinel sign as well function of the nerve involved can be looked for. The PSSD machine is a valuable tool to monitor nerve healing. The PSSD machine provides 1-point and 2-point pressure and discrimination values that can be tracked. If there is not more than 10% improvement in the sensation of the affected nerve and no significant pain relief with 3 months of conservative therapy, then surgery should be considered. Every patient is different and other medical issues may influence the decision to proceed with surgery or continue with conservative therapy. The use of sclerosing alcohol injections and cryotherapy are intended to destroy nerve tissue and, once this has been done, ongoing treatment is limited to further destructive techniques. Looking at the typical treatment of an intermetatarsal nerve entrapment, where patients may receive a series of alcohol injections or steroids, these patients often go on to have a neurectomy, which is mostly successful but, when not successful, can lead to a stump neuroma with terrible consequences that require a much more involved treatment plan usually involving surgery of the plantar arch of the foot. It is the experience of one of the authors (PJB) that, in most cases, decompression is the preferred treatment over any destructive nerve procedure when there is no evidence of any true nerve injury.

The genesis of this author's (PJB's) interest in the diagnosis and treatment of SFN entrapment evolved from seeing certain patients with foot pain that was difficult to successfully treat. As an example, a patient presents with generalized lateral column pain or dorsolateral foot pain. It was usually exacerbated by squeezing the foot from side to side and bothered the patient with ambulation. The patient had symptoms localized to the dorsolateral aspect of the foot, as a result of entrapment of 1 of the branches of the SFN, which had a separate fascial sheath between the anterior and lateral compartments, which was alleviated by means of external neurolysis. This was reported by Rosson and Dellon in 2005.[5]

This commentary focuses on the entrapment of the SFN. The author (PJB) has operated on 35 cases of SFN entrapment over the past 4 years, with duration of follow-up of at least 1 year. At the authors' center, close track is kept of the results of each particular nerve condition and the results of the interventions. Successful surgical intervention is defined as a 50% decrease in subjective pain, as defined in the Visual Analog Scale 10-cm pain scale, combined with patient indication that if the symptoms were the same, the patient would undergo the same surgery again. The current incidence of success is 92% over a 4-year observation period. The purpose of this commentary is to inform readers about this pathology and for them to be able diagnose this often overlooked nerve pathology and provide appropriate treatment or proper referral to a peripheral nerve specialist. It is important not to undertake any peripheral nerve surgery without proper training and experience.

ANATOMY OF THE SUPERFICIAL FIBULAR NERVE

The SFN supplies motor innervation to the fibularis longus and fibularis brevis muscles as well as cutaneous innervation to the anteroinferior portion of the leg and much of dorsum of the foot and toes. The SFN emerges as a terminal branch at the bifurcation of the common fibular nerve in the popliteal fossa, near the fibular head. After supplying the fibularis musculature, the SFN typically passes inferiorly in the lateral leg, between the fibularis longus and the anterior crural intermuscular septum. In 23% to 27% of the population, the SFN may travel in the anterior compartment of the leg rather than the lateral compartment.[6,7] In this case, the SFN may also provide muscular branches to the extensor hallucis longus muscle.[8,9] Approximately 7.7 cm from the intermalleolar line, the SFN passes between the fibularis longus and the extensor digitorum longus and pierces the crural fascia.[8] There is variability in where it becomes superficial through the fascia. The SFN then splits into a medial dorsal cutaneous nerve (MDCN) and an intermediate dorsal cutaneous nerve (IDCN); a lateral dorsal cutaneous nerve also exists as a branch from the sural nerve. Alternatively, in approximately 28% of the population, the SFN may split into terminal branches while still deep to the crural fascia.[8,9] In this case, the MDCN typically emerges from the crural fascia, approximately 8.1 cm proximal to the intermalleolar line, whereas the IDCN emerges 2.6 cm more distally.[8] Regardless of its point of emergence, the MDCN crosses anterior to the talocrural joint, equidistant from the medial and lateral malleoli, and bifurcates into dorsal digital nerves, supplying parts of digits 1 to 3.[9] The IDCN also crosses the anterior of the talocrural joint at approximately one-third the distance from the lateral malleolus to the medial malleolus and branches to provide dorsal branches to digits 3 to 5 as well as a cutaneous branch to the lateral malleolus.[9] In rare instances, the MDCN or IDCN may be absent. When this occurs, branches of the saphenous or sural nerves cover the cutaneous innervation, respectively[9] (**Fig. 1**).

It is important to appreciate the variable course of the SFN and its branches for the purpose of graft harvesting and to avoid iatrogenic injury. The MDCN and IDCN are endangered during the creation of anterolateral ports for arthroscopic procedures. Because the common site of anterolateral portal placement is along the lateral border of the fibularis tertius tendon or extensor digitorum longus tendon,[10,11] the IDCN is at greater risk. To minimize the risk of damage, it may be possible to visualize the SFN and its terminal branches. In some patients, the SFN is visible on plantar flexion (approximately 10°) and inversion.[11] As the foot is moved from plantarflexion, through neutral, and into dorsiflexion (approximately 5°), the SFN and its terminal branches displace laterally by a few millimeters.[10] Visualization of the SFN is further accentuated by flexion of the fourth digit,[10] and transillumination may also enhance visualization.[11] Alternatively, the course of the SFN can be traced with ultrasonography if needed.

DIAGNOSIS OF SUPERFICIAL FIBULAR NERVE ENTRAPMENT

How can the correct diagnosis of an SFN injury or entrapment be made? Making a correct diagnosis of SFN pathology can be a difficult task. The symptoms tend to mimic other diagnoses but a thorough history and examination point surgeons in the right direction. Initially many patients with this type of nerve pain have sustained a traumatic injury to the lower leg, ankle, or foot that directly crushes, stretches, or tears the nerve trunk at the site of injury or additionally at a more proximal or distal location. If the mechanical force of this particular injury was sufficient enough to stretch or tear ankle ligaments, muscles, or tendons; fracture the fibula and/or tibia; or tear the syndesmotic ankle ligament, then there was more than enough energy to damage the relatively unprotected peripheral nerve(s). This injury could have occurred months or years prior to a patient seeking professional care, so it is important to document any trauma as far back as possible.

A patient's occupation can also play a role in making the diagnosis. For example, dancers who frequently plantarflex and invert their ankle, in particular ballerinas en pointe, are prone to SFN entrapment and injury. Most prevalently, the common

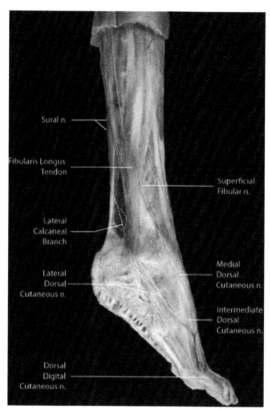

Fig. 1. Cadaveric prosection of the lateral leg showing the neuroanatomy of the SFN and the intermediate and MDCNs and the sural nerve. n., nerve.

inversion ankle sprain (contraction) or contusion to the anterolateral aspect of the leg blunt compression is responsible for entrapment of the SFN and/or its branches.[1] The inversion injury involves high-velocity, rapid stretching of the nerve trunk in the leg where it emerges through the fascia (often referred to as Henry's hiatus) as it exits the muscle compartment through the deep fascia. At this level, there can be direct trauma to the more distal divisions of the medial and IDCNs, traversing distally over the anterior lateral ankle and dorsal foot surfaces. Direct contusion to SFN trunk occurs most typically in athletes involved in field sports, such as soccer, field hockey, lacrosse, and football. Frequently, in softball and volleyball, players are injured when the ball strikes the lateral leg, resulting in contusion, disruption in the fascia, and herniation of the nerve into the subcutaneous layer (**Fig. 2**). It is also common to see these injuries in martial arts at any level of competition or training.

Anatomic anomaly, such as muscle herniation, can also result in or predispose to SFN entrapment and this condition was described by Yang,[12] who reported successful treatment of the entrapment with external neurolysis and treatment. Seddon type 1 stretch injuries (without neural tear) represent more than 95% of this injury pattern and Seddon type 2 partial tear injuries are less than 5% that are clinically encountered.[13] As can be seen, the SFN or its branches are vulnerable to injury in association with surgical repair of ruptured ankle ligaments, peroneal tendons, fixation of fibular fractures, and ankle arthroscopy using trocars placed through soft tissue portals. Chronic

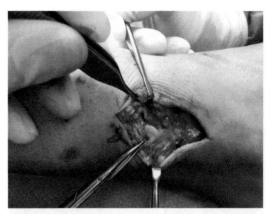

Fig. 2. Intraoperative view of the distal branch of the SFN, which has formed as neuroma in continuity, as it herniates through the deep fascia in the lateral compartment.

postinjury inflammatory changes, which can develop in response to a wide range of pathologies, such as blunt or sectioning injuries, hematoma, cast immobilization, connective tissue disease, or infection, can lead to the formation of adhesions that entrap the SFN trunk in its adjacent soft tissues.

Clinical examination of a patient with a suspected SFN problem entails the typical elements of lower extremity sensory and motor testing, including assessment of 2-point discrimination, vibratory sensation, monofilament esthesiometer sensation, manual muscle strength testing, assessment of deep tendon reflexes at the Achilles and patellar levels, superficial reflex assessment, and evaluation of the straight leg raise test and slump test. Focal palpation and manipulation of the suspected nerve trunk, with identification of a positive or negative Tinel sign, is also documented.

The use of diagnostic ultrasound enables visually identifying the nerves in the compartments of the leg. MRI neurography has allowed seeing areas of compression along the course of the entire peripheral nerve (although it is expensive and has limited availability).[14,15] Once damage to the SFN and/or its branches is suspected, the authors advise systematically isolating the nerve and mark this out in the patient chart, noting the exact location of the most painful site as well as any Tinel sign and the distribution of radiation of the sign. For example, documenting can be as follows: +Tinel's sign 12 cm proximal to fibular malleolus and 2 cm lateral to tibial spine with radiation to the fourth metatarsal. The next step is performing diagnostic (and therapeutic) nerve blocks using only small amounts of lidocaine to attempt to temporarily relieve the patient of symptoms. It is important to know the anatomy when doing blocks so the responses can be interpreted. Individual responses to these diagnostic blocks need to be correlated with a physician's knowledge of the variations in SFN branch patterns to develop a proper diagnosis. This helps determine if there are anatomic variations of the SFN present or additional peripheral sensory nerves that are involved.

Regarding peripheral nerve blockade with the use of a local anesthetic agent, it is important to note the position in the leg; the nerve may be deep or superficial to the crural fascia and the patient may need to be injected twice, with documentation of each response in the patient chart. The first injection is infiltrated in the subcutaneous tissue and if the patient does not describe greater than 75% relief after a few minutes, then a second injection result is given deep to the deep fascia layer. Placement of this second injection can be aided by ultrasound guidance. Once the documentation of the second injection results is complete, the appropriate treatment is determined. It may be helpful to repeat the diagnostic nerve block on another visit to confirm the response to the injection and to better allow the patient to understand what can be anticipated should surgery be undertaken. After blockade of the SFN, extensive sensory anesthesia, as well as autonomic moor dysfunction, should be observed. If the first web space is spared and the patient's symptoms are adequately relieved, then it is unlikely that the deep peroneal nerve is involved in any of the patient's symptoms. It is also important to determine whether or not peripheral neuropathy (polyneuritis) is present and to distinguish it from a localized peripheral nerve entrapment (mononeuritis). This distinction can be made in several ways, including the use of a PSSD machine[16] or, if that is not available, then a 2-point tactile discriminator (**Fig. 3**) suffices.

SURGICAL DECOMPRESSION OF THE SUPERFICIAL FIBULAR NERVE

After determining via diagnostic blocks and clinical examination that there is an entrapment of 1 or more branches of the SFN, then it should first be explained to the patient that the success rate of the decompression is approximately 85%[17–19] if diagnosed correctly. The authors believe that it is important to explain to patients that every person does not have the same "peripheral nerve anatomy" and that even though the diagnostic block and the subsequent surgical decompression were indicated and properly executed, it is possible that other peripheral nerves contribute to the symptoms and that this contribution by another nerve or nerves could be unmasked by the surgery may require further surgery. Preoperative documentation should be made of a patient's maximum point of pain and Tinel sign as well as the distribution of the Tinel sign, because these are the strongest indicators of the specific nerve that requires decompression. When tapped percutaneously, the patient experiences pain and/or parasthesias at the sight of percussion or usually distally in the anatomic distribution of the nerve. Sometimes the parasthesias radiates in the area of another named nerve, which can be confusing, and indicates a possible anatomic anomaly. Knowledge of the location of the Tinel sign enables surgeons to localize the incision over the most likely area of entrapment (**Fig. 4**). The authors have also found that perioperative use of drugs, such as gabapentin, desipramine, topiramate, vitamin C, and topical analgesic compounds, can be useful. These medications not only help

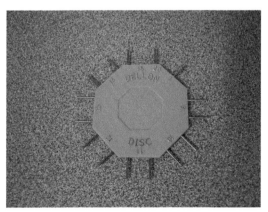

Fig. 3. Diagram of 2-point discriminator. (*Courtesy of* US Neurologicals, LLC, Poulsbo, WA; with permission.)

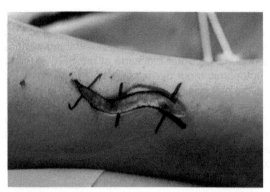

Fig. 4. Typical 6-cm incision to allow access to the SFN in the anterior and lateral compartment of the leg. It is centered approximately 11 cm to 12 cm above the ankle joint.

patients prior to the decision to operate but also help during the recovery process, and in some patients these medications are continued indefinitely.

On the day of the surgery, the patient can be met in the preoperative holding area and the area to be decompressed confirmed and marked. Video 1 shows the decompression of the nerve with use of amniotic tissue graft.

The patient is then taken to the operating room and placed on the operating table in the supine position; a well-padded thigh tourniquet is applied at the surgeon's discretion. The surgery could be performed with or without use of tourniquet hemostasis. If using a thigh tourniquet, then it is strongly encouraged to use general anesthesia because any tourniquet time of more than 20 minutes starts to cause painful ischemia and requires more anesthesia. The surgery can also be done easily with a spinal anesthesia without the side effects or risks of general anesthesia. Intravenous sedation is another choice but it is the authors' (PJB's) preference to avoid it because the other options are better tolerated. A superficial local anesthetic block is used to anesthetize the area of the planned dissection and in this case it is where the SFN emerges through the deep fascia and becomes subcutaneous. It is important to avoid excessive volume of local anesthetic so as not to obliterate the underlying anatomy. Bipolar cautery is used to coagulate any small vessels as well as fascia. Careful skin retraction is carried out using double skin hooks and meticulous tissue handling is always observed. To adequately decompress the SFN, the author (PJB) prefers a lazy-S type of incision, approximately 5 cm to 6 cm in length, although this can be extended at the surgeon's discretion and 2 or 3 smaller incisions can be made to provide a more thorough decompression if needed. After opening the skin, sharp and blunt dissection methods using tenotomy scissors as well as diligent use of a wet sponge to help spread the adipose tissue are applied. The nerve(s) usually are encountered below the crural fascia at this level, although it is certainly possible to encounter a branch or 2 in the subcutaneous layer. Usually tendon and nerve can be seen through the crural fascia and these structures can guide the placement of the deep incision. A #15 blade is then used to perforate the deep/crural fascia after which the crural fascia is incised along the course of the nerve to expose it. Bipolar cautery is used to cauterize the margins of the deep fascia to avoid postoperative scar complications, because the fascia is a source of scar tissue that could adhere to the decompressed nerve trunk. After incising the crural fascia, access is gained to both the lateral (peroneal) and anterior muscle compartments of the leg; then careful inspection is carried to identify the

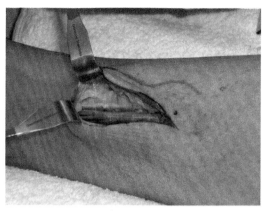

Fig. 5. Intraoperative incision showing the SFN decompressed as it splits into its terminal named branches.

SFB and all its branches. It is important to look with in the septum between the 2 compartments because a branch of the nerve can be located there as well (**Fig. 5**); this maneuver is demonstrated in Video 1, which displays a patient who had the SFN entrapped within a separate fascial tunnel in the anterior compartment of the leg.

The fundamental maneuver required to effectively decompress the SFN and its branches is external neurolysis, and it is important to dissect both proximal and distal along the course of the nerve(s) until the trunks are no longer visually compressed. It is helpful to have an assistant use a deep retractor to elevate the skin so that the surgeon can look down the tunnel and make sure that no gross visual entrapment persists. Distally, the surgeon should be able to see the nerve split into the IDCN and the MDCN as they course toward the foot. Once all of the branches have been inspected and freed from any entrapment, any tissue that could produce scar tissue is electrocauterized with the bipolar unit after which copious lavage is performed (**Fig. 6**). Opening the anterior and lateral compartments is essentially performing fasciotomies of the respective compartments. This is especially important in the clinical setting of exercised induced chronic compartment syndrome. After SFN decompression and wound lavage, a cocktail of local anesthetic and dexamethasone phosphate is used to bathe the exposed nerve trunk to prolong local anesthesia and diminish immediate inflammation and fibroproliferation. This advised unless using any biologics, such as amniotic tissue graft or fluid (which is the author's [PJB's] preferred choice). If a tourniquet was used and there are any doubts about hemostasis, the tourniquet should be deflated prior to closure. Closure of the wound does not include the reapproximation of the crural fascia. The subcutaneous tissue is reapproximated with a few 4-0 poligle-caprone 25 sutures just enough to keep tension off the skin. The skin is closed with suture of surgeon's choice and a Jones compression dressing is applied.

After the operation, the patient is encouraged to move the toes and ankle as much as desired while keeping the leg elevated for the first 48 hours. It is generally inappropriate to immobilize any extremity after any decompression of an in-continuity nerve trunk. The patient can walk up to 30 to 40 feet per hour for the first week then double that for the second week. The patient can walk as much as can be tolerated after 3 weeks as long as there is no significant swelling. Postoperative physical therapy is used as soon as possible after the first week, and aqua therapy is recommended after the skin sutures have been removed approximately 2 to 3 weeks after surgery. Nerve gliding techniques can also be helpful and should be instituted as soon as possible. It

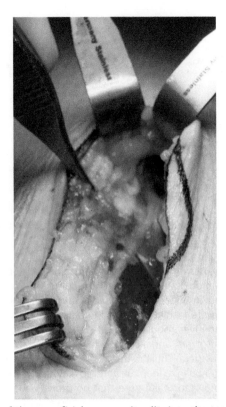

Fig. 6. Close-up view of the superficial nerve as it splits into the terminal branches.

typically takes up to 4 to 6 weeks after the surgery before the patient can resume full activity without restrictions.

Achieving a successful outcome is predicated on performing the correct surgery and setting expectations accordingly. The generally accepted incidence of success after decompression of an in-continuity SFN trunk is approximately 85%.[17–20] The definition of success must also be discussed with each patient. Many factors come into play, including but not limited to chronic use of pain medication, past medical history, history of depression, history of injury, smoking history, and patient's desired functional level, to name a few. Failure of any decompression should be looked at closely and the surgeon needs to evaluate carefully why the surgery may have failed. The longer a patient has had the condition then the less likely the chance of a positive outcome. It is also important to determine if there are any other peripheral nerve contributions to a patient's pain that may have been missed, including more proximal pathology, such as lumbosacral pathology. Any central nervous system issues also must be ruled out, especially a patient who may have centralized nerve pain. In cases of chronic nerve pain, the peripheral nerve problem can become centralized and this needs to be handled in a much different manner and requires a multifaceted approach. In cases of the SFN, the sural nerve may be contributing a branch or even be the source of the problem. It is important to make clear to patients preoperatively that everyone is not neurologically wired the same. The analogy of a house that was wired back in the 1960s works well when discussing variation in nerve distribution. An electrician assessing the house without being able to see the specific mechanical blueprints may have an idea of how things are wired but would not actually know until physically inspecting the actual wires. This analogy is helpful in explaining the surgery and its possible outcomes prior to undertaking decompression of the SFN. As discussed previously, reasons that these types of surgeries can fail is if the pain has become centralized, as is the case in many patients with chronic pain. In these cases, comanagement with a pain management specialist is required and the care of an experienced biopsychologist can be beneficial. The incidence of surgical success after decompression dramatically decreases in the face of centralized pain. Another facet of managing a patient with nerve pain is perioperative management. Still further, and as discussed previously, adjunct use of medications, such as gabapentin and topical analgesic compounds, can be useful in the preoperative and postoperative decompression period. Overall, a team approach to the peripheral nerve patient provides patients with the highest degree of success. This team includes anesthesia, pain management, psychology, physical therapy, and the surgeon. With proper training and experience, peripheral nerve surgeons can make an accurate and timely diagnosis and properly execute external neurolysis and successful decompression of the SFN (or any other nerve in the lower extremity).

In summary, the author (PJB) has commented on the approach to identification and treatment of entrapment of the SFN. This is an important topic of discussion for foot and ankle surgeons, because overlooking the diagnosis can lead to permanent nerve damage. The aim is to inform the readers of this pathology and remind them to consider it and not overlook the possibility of this condition as a cause of foot and ankle symptomology, because early diagnosis and treatment are, in the opinion of the author (PJB), crucial to avoidance of permanent nerve damage. Not every foot and ankle surgeon is interested in undertaking peripheral nerve surgery, and appropriate referral to a surgeon who specializes in treatment of the peripheral nerve can be helpful in making the proper diagnosis and receiving appropriate care, nonsurgical or otherwise. The Association of Extremity Nerve Surgeons has published guidelines on the diagnosis and treatment of peripheral nerve problems in the lower extremity, which readers can use as a reference and which can be found on their Web site: www.AENS.US.

SUPPLEMENTARY DATA

Supplementary data related to this article can be found at http://dx.doi.org/10.1016/j.cpm.2015.12.007.

REFERENCES

1. Kernohan J, Levack B, Wilson JN. Entrapment of the superficial peroneal nerve. Three case reports. J Bone Joint Surg Br 1985;67:60–1.
2. Styf J. Entrapment of the superficial peroneal nerve. Diagnosis and results of decompression. J Bone Joint Surg Br 1989;71:131–5.
3. Donovan A, Rosenberg ZS, Cavalcanti CF. MR imaging of entrapment neuropathies of the lower extremity. Part 2. The knee, leg, ankle, and foot. Radiographics 2010;30:1001–19.
4. Anandkumar S. Physical therapy management of entrapment of the superficial peroneal nerve in the lower leg: a case report. Physiother Theory Pract 2012;28:552–61.
5. Rosson GD, Dellon AL. Superficial peroneal nerve anatomic variability changes surgical technique. Clin Orthop Relat Res 2005;438:248–52.

6. Barrett SL, Dellon AL, Rosson GD, et al. Superficial peroneal nerve (superficial fibularis nerve): the clinical implications of anatomic variability. J Foot Ankle Surg 2006;45:174–6.

7. Canella C, Demondion X, Guillin R, et al. Anatomic study of the superficial peroneal nerve using sonography. AJR Am J Roentgenol 2009;193:174–9.

8. Agthong S, Huanmanop T, Sasivongsbhakdi T, et al. Anatomy of the superficial peroneal nerve related to the harvesting for nerve graft. Surg Radiol Anat 2008; 30:145–8.

9. Blair JM, Botte MJ. Surgical anatomy of the superficial peroneal nerve in the ankle and foot. Clin Orthop Relat Res 1994;305:229–38.

10. Stephens MM, Kelly PM. Fourth toe flexion sign: a new clinical sign for identification of the superficial peroneal nerve. Foot Ankle Int 2000;21:860–3.

11. De Leeuw PA, Golano P, Sierevelt IN, et al. The course of the superficial peroneal nerve in relation to the ankle position: anatomical study with ankle arthroscopic implications. Knee Surg Sports Traumatol Arthrosc 2010;18:612–7.

12. Yang LJ, Gala VC, McGillicuddy JE. Superficial peroneal nerve syndrome: an unusual nerve entrapment. Case report. J Neurosurg 2006;104:820–3.

13. Seddon HJ. A classification of nerve injuries. Br Med J 1942;2:237–9.

14. Pham M, Baumer T, Bendszus M. Peripheral nerves and plexus: imaging by MR-neurography and high-resolution ultrasound. Curr Opin Neurol 2014;27:370–9.

15. Aagaard BD, Maravilla KR, Kliot M. Magnetic resonance neurography: magnetic resonance imaging of peripheral nerves. Neuroimaging Clin N Am 2001;11: 131–46.

16. Tassler PL, Dellon AL. Pressure perception in the normal lower extremity and in the tarsal tunnel syndrome. Muscle Nerve 1996;19:285–9.

17. Valdivia JM, Dellon AL, Weinand ME, et al. Surgical treatment of peripheral neuropathy: outcomes from 100 consecutive decompressions. J Am Podiatr Med Assoc 2005;95:451–4.

18. Siemionow M, Alghoulk M, Molski M, et al. Clinical outcome of peripheral nerve decompression in diabetic and nondiabetic peripheral neuropathy. Ann Plast Surg 2006;57:385–90.

19. Zhang W, Li S, Zheng X. Evaluation of the clinical efficacy of multiple lower extremity nerve decompression in diabetic peripheral neuropathy. J Neurol Surg A Cent Eur Neurosurg 2013;74:96–100.

20. Aszmann OC, Kress KM, Dellon AL. Results of decompression of peripheral nerves in diabetics: a prospective, blinded study. Plast Reconstr Surg 2000; 106:816–22.

Intraoperative Nerve Monitoring During Nerve Decompression Surgery in the Lower Extremity

James C. Anderson, DPM[a],*, Dwayne S. Yamasaki, PhD[b]

KEYWORDS

- Nerve decompression • Intraoperative neural monitor • Lower extremity
- Peripheral neuropathy

KEY POINTS

- Intraoperative neurophysiologic monitoring (IONM) can be helpful for educating the patient and improving the quality of services provided when nerve decompression is done.
- IONM can give the surgeon better feedback regarding the amount of decompression to be done while performing a neurolysis procedure.
- IONM can give the surgeon objective information regarding changes in nerve function for better medical documentation.
- IONM can provide objective data to further research regarding outcomes of nerve decompressions in the lower extremity.
- IONM can assist the doctor in economizing surgical time when attempting to localize nerves in challenging surgical cases.

 Video content accompanies this article at http://www.podiatric.theclinics.com

INTRODUCTION

It has been estimated that 15–20 million people over the age of 40 suffer from peripheral neuropathy in the United States, many of whom have diabetic neuropathy.[1] Approximately 50% of people with diabetes have some form of neuropathy and those with diabetic neuropathy are at higher risk of disease progression leading to gangrene

Disclosure Statement: J.C. Anderson has no financial disclosures or conflicts of interest; D.S. Yamasaki is an employee of Medtronic but Medtronic had no influence on the intraoperative paper.
[a] Anderson Podiatry Center for Nerve Pain, 1355 Riverside Avenue, Fort Collins, CO 80524, USA;
[b] Medtronic, Jacksonville, FL, USA
* Corresponding author.
E-mail address: JAnderson@ANDERSONPODIATRYCENTER.COM

Clin Podiatr Med Surg 33 (2016) 255–266
http://dx.doi.org/10.1016/j.cpm.2015.12.003
0891-8422/16/$ – see front matter © 2016 Elsevier Inc. All rights reserved.

podiatric.theclinics.com

and amputation.[2] These estimates do not include the 38% of the US population who are considered prediabetic. Therefore, between 49% and 52% of the United States population is considered diabetic or prediabetic, and many of these individuals are undiagnosed.[3] Although the most common cause of neuropathy is diabetes, many other individuals suffer from nondiabetic neuropathy. Most of these nondiabetic patients have been diagnosed with idiopathic polyneuropathy. Most of the patients undergoing decompression procedures are nondiabetic among this population.

The concept of nerve decompression for diabetic neuropathy was first described in 1992[4] and for nondiabetic neuropathy in 2006.[5] Decompression for diabetic neuropathy was first reported in the podiatric literature in 2003.[6] More recent studies have been published indicating the significance of decreased rates of amputation and ulcers in diabetics.[7–9] In 2014, Zhong and colleagues[10] published findings showing that in a 1526 subject study many subjects had significant improvement in their nerve conduction velocity as well as their quantitative sensory testing a year and a half after decompression surgery. This group demonstrated similar improvement in 560 subjects at 18 months, in addition to improved motor function and skin ulcer healing.[11]

Despite the published evidence, nerve decompression surgery as a treatment of diabetic and nondiabetic neuropathy still remains controversial. Intraoperative neurophysiologic monitoring (IONM) is useful for an array of applications, not the least of which is establishing more objective evidence on physiologic change to nerve function. This objective measure will help researchers and clinicians better understand the physiologic changes that occur as a result of nerve decompression surgery among those with peripheral neuropathy.

IONM is used routinely in thyroid and fascial surgery,[12–15] spinal surgery,[16] and otologic skull-based procedures.[17] For all of these procedures, IONM is used to monitor the integrity of the nerves at risk during the procedure. IONM, as presented here, is used not only to monitor nerve integrity but also to determine if nerve decompression improves nerve function. The results also provide additional information to share with the patient.

The common fibular nerve innervates the dorsum of the foot and passes through the anterior lateral compartment, whereas the tibial nerve innervates the plantar aspect of the foot and passes through both the tarsal tunnel and soleal sling. Both of these nerves have a detectable number of motor branches and their function can be measured during a surgical decompression. It is understood that the superficial fibular and deep fibular nerves have motor branches; however, the muscle components are small and it is not practical to monitor them intraoperatively. Because IONM records evoked potentials in muscle, its use is limited to nerves where a significant number of motor branches are located. However, it is not necessary for the patient to experience significant motor impairment for improvement to be noted. This is because it is presumed that the same compression that is causing dysfunction of the motor fascicles is also causing dysfunction to the sensory fascicles. Therefore, improvement in evoked potentials as recorded during IONM will also benefit patients suffering from burning, tingling, and numbness; which are commonly affected sensory modalities.

Introducing nerve monitoring to the surgical arena will often cause a skeptical physician to consider the added time to the surgery as a serious dilemma. However, as the physician becomes more efficient, the added time is minimal (approximately 5–10 minutes) and the benefits outweigh the risks associated with a slightly longer surgery. The following protocol is a very basic overview. Over time, not only should the time it takes to perform IONM be reduced but improvements in consistency should also be improved. This should result in IONM becoming a standard protocol in decompression surgeries. Considering the advantages of nerve monitoring, the following aspects should be considered: improved patient education, improvement in surgical technique and potential results, improvement in documentation, data collection for research purposes, and improvement in the surgeon's ability to locate the nerve to be decompressed.

IONM can be used with great accuracy to identify the location to begin the decompression via the stimulating electrode. Because nerve decompression may be a new technique for many surgeons, IONM is a particularly useful exercise to apply while learning the procedure to help the surgeon become more proficient at performing decompressions. Many lower extremity surgeons are familiar with the anatomy of the tarsal tunnel because this may have been part of their formal training. However, the soleal sling and common fibular anatomy will be unfamiliar for most podiatric surgeons. Practicing IONM in the early phase of the surgeon's technical training will also instill confidence by helping to locate the nerve and by identifying what was, or was not, nervous tissue. This may particularly be the case with the common fibular nerve. The concern of drop foot as an adverse effect of surgery is a motivating factor for nerve monitoring. A revision surgery is another example of when nerve monitoring is useful for localization of the nerve. A revision surgery often results in mistaking fibrotic scar tissue for nervous tissue. Applying IONM can aid in overcoming this obstacle because scar tissue will not produce evoked potentials, whereas the nervous tissue will. This method can help locate the nerve even when it may not be macroscopically visible or other localization methods fail. Additionally, IONM can be useful to avoid trauma to other nearby vital structures, such as blood vessels. This is particularly true with decompression of the soleal sling because the tibial artery and vein of the lower limb lie in this area. For instance, during decompression of the tibial nerve throughout the soleal sling, the stimulating probe is used to help guide the dissection.

The IONM technique can also provide documentation of nerve function at the completion of the surgery, with improvement noted in most cases. Surgeons are formally trained to take intraoperative fluoroscopy during orthopedic procedures as a way to document the results of the surgery before the patient leaves the operating room and is transferred to recovery. This same principle should apply to nerve surgeries. In most cases, the surgeon should be able to appreciate improved nerve function when comparing the predecompression evoked potential value to the postdecompression value. It should be noted that in cases in which nerve monitoring did not show improvement it does not mean that the patient did not improve. It should also be noted that improved muscle contraction in the muscle group being stimulated may also be observed in the operating room. This may be a secondary way to ensure that no damage was done to the involved nerve branch. This may also be documented in the patient's operation report.

Patient education is very important because patients can be shown the results immediately following their surgery while still in the recovery area. Many patients are anxious to hear how successful the surgery was and this can provide them with that information. An educated and satisfied patient can then serve as a source to inform others, as well as their primary care physicians, of the success of their surgery. Therefore, it should be considered standard practice to follow this same protocol in regard to what was done in the surgical arena with a patient's nerves.

If the surgeon is interested in research, IONM can be useful in gaining objective information from the surgery. The more surgeons are engaged in clinical research, the more we will understand which demographic is benefiting more from the surgeries, and the more effective we will be at applying and executing the procedures.

IONM can serve as a tool to show the physiologic benefits associated with nerve decompression as a treatment of neuropathy. Contemporary physicians practice outcome-based medicine and, with objective documentation acquired from IONM, physicians will be confident in the medicine that they are practicing. This IONM documentation is also useful in reassuring patients about the benefits of nerve decompression from an unbiased perspective.

The intraoperative monitoring technique also provides the surgeon with feedback indicating how effective the decompression has been thus far and if to continue decompressing. In some cases, this feedback will indicate that the surgeon should conduct a more thorough neurolysis of the nerve. While the surgeon is performing the neurolysis on a particular tunnel, it is necessary to periodically stimulate the associated nerve to provide the feedback about nerve function as the decompression proceeds. For the less experienced surgeon, this information may also give feedback about how aggressive the neurolysis should be. The feedback may also indicate at which point during the decompression neurolysis is complete and additional decompression would not yield any additional benefit.

PROCEDURE

So how is nerve monitoring done? It must be emphasized that the information presented here is a very general overview. Presented here are the methods for IONM at the tarsal tunnel, the common fibular, and the soleal sling using the NIM 3.0 Nerve Monitoring System (Medtronic, plc, Jacksonville, FL, USA) (Videos 1 and 2). Before nerve decompression is begun, the following guidelines for setup should be considered. If an ankle or thigh tourniquet is used it may serve as another site of compression and nerve ischemia, and may affect the IONM recordings and, therefore, the procedures are best performed without a tourniquet. It is presumed the external compression will decrease blood flow and oxygen to the nerve tissue, thereby affecting the status of nerve function. Intraoperatively, it has been observed that if a tourniquet is used for around 30 minutes or more this can have a significant impact on the IONM recordings. In an 11 subject pilot study in which IONM was performed both before and after nerve decompression, there was a trend for a geometric drop in percent change in electromyographic (EMG) amplitude with increased tourniquet time (Video 3). At 14 minutes of tourniquet time the average change in EMG was 538%, whereas at 36 minutes the average change was 68.5% (a drop of 31.5% from baseline).[18] This is consistent with other reports showing ischemic effects on nerve function starting at 25 to 30 minutes.[19] How significant the impact is when tourniquet time is less than 30 minutes has not been determined. If nerve function is impaired, such as when a tourniquet is used, it may be more difficult to achieve an evoked potential. Therefore, more current will need to be applied to get the muscles being recorded to respond. Between the initial recording, before decompression is done, and the final recording, when decompression is completed, a decreased response may be noted. When the common fibular nerve is monitored, the tibialis anterior and peroneus longus muscles are recorded (Fig. 1). When tarsal tunnel or soleal sling surgery is performed, the abductor hallucis and abductor digiti quinti are recorded (Fig. 2). This is accomplished by placement of bipolar needle electrodes in each of these muscles (see Fig. 1A) and recording evoked potentials on the NIM monitor (see Fig. 1B). Electrode placement in the abductor hallucis is 1 to 2 cm distal to the navicular tuberosity on the medial aspect of the arch. The abductor digiti quinti placement is midway between the fifth metatarsal head and the styloid process on the lateral plantar side of the foot. The location for the tibialis anterior muscle is 4 finger widths (approximately 7.6 cm) distal to the tibial tuberosity and approximately 1 cm lateral to the crest of the tibia. For the peroneus longus, the electrode is placed 3 finger widths (approximately 5.7 cm) distal

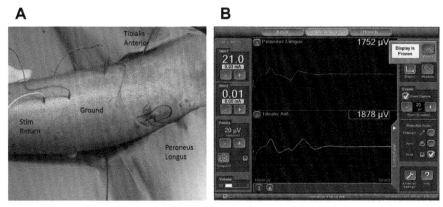

Fig. 1. Common fibular setup. (*A*) Placement of color-coded electrodes. The red electrodes are inserted into the tibialis anterior, the blue electrodes are inserted into the peroneus longus, the ground electrode is between the stimulus return (STIM), and the recording electrodes in an area away from the surgical site. (*B*) Color-coded electrodes relay to the NIM monitor showing the evoked potentials (μV) in the peroneus longus and tibialis anterior.

to the head of the fibula and 1 cm anterior to the fibula. It is recommended to bury the needle recording electrode in the muscle so the hub is resting against the skin (**Fig. 3**). Some surgeons prefer the technique of bending the needles at the level of the hub once the needles are in the muscle so the hub sits parallel to the skin. Sterile adhesive (ie, Tegaderm) may also be used to adhere the electrode to the skin. The goal in both setups is to avoid movement of the electrode once recording begins. As the muscle is stimulated and contracture occurs, the needle electrodes may move from a deep to a more superficial position because of the mechanical effect of the muscle on the electrodes. It is important to keep the same electrode positioning in the muscle once the recording protocol has begun. The nerve may be stimulated with currents ranging between 0 mA and 30 mA. When stimulating at higher current levels (ie, >20 mA), use a stimulating probe with a diameter ≥1.0 mm in order to minimize the current density and potential tissue injury. In addition to the visual display on the NIM 3.0, a sound

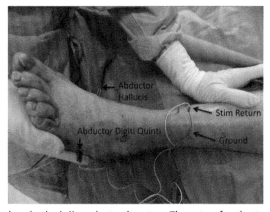

Fig. 2. Tarsal tunnel and soleal sling electrode setup. The setup for the tarsal tunnel and soleal sling is similar to that of the common fibular.

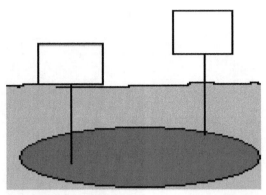

Fig. 3. Placement of the recording electrode. Muscle contracture during stimulation may push the electrode out of the muscle. Observe the electrodes while stimulating to make sure the same depth is maintained or use sterile adhesive to tape them to the leg.

is emitted with a higher volume indicating higher evoked potential amplitudes. Each recording electrode in the muscle is color coded to match the color on the monitor of that muscle's response (see **Fig. 1**). Also, each channel has a different pitch that can be heard from the speaker on the monitor. This allows the surgeon to know how each channel and/or muscle is responding without the need to look at the monitoring screen. The evoked potentials recorded from the needle electrodes are presented in microvolts. If more nerve damage is present, it may be necessary to use more stimulation to get adequate evoked potentials in the muscle group being monitored. Placement of the electrode in the muscle may also need to be adjusted.

The current protocol is as follows. When dissection is down to the soft tissues structures that form the tunnel, the stimulating electrode may be placed on the overlying tissue to help localize the nerve. The location of the area to be tested is proximal to the anatomic site of compression. Once the nerve is located, a small 0.5 cm window is made through the tissue for placement of the stimulating electrode on the nerve. The surgeon then maps the fascicular topography of the nerve by stimulating various sides of the nerve while monitoring the evoked EMG of the target muscles (**Fig. 4**). Once the locations of the desired fascicles (ie, those innervating the monitored muscles) have been located and everything is ready for testing, the stimulus current is set to zero.

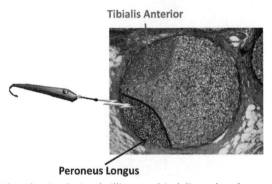

Fig. 4. Nerve fascicles. The simulation (milliampere) is delivered to the nerve fascicle and the corresponding evoked potential (microvolts) is displayed on the neural monitor.

The surgeon then maintains the stimulating electrode in the same position on the nerve (ie, both along the length and side of the nerve). The amperage is gradually increased until the first evoked potential, or threshold, is recorded. This is then recorded as the initial response. The current, as well as the evoked potential amplitude, is then recorded (saved) on the monitor. The current is gradually increased, maintaining the same position of the electrode on the nerve until the evoked potential values plateau. The stimulus current and evoked potential amplitudes are again recorded and this will serve as the baseline recording. When the evoked potentials have plateaued, this indicates that all the fascicles of the nerve being stimulated are fully saturated with current (**Fig. 5**). This process is then repeated with the other muscle being tested. The predecompression nerve function is assessed for both muscles (**Fig. 6**). After determining the baseline evoked potential for each muscle, as well as the corresponding amperage to achieve it, the nerve decompression is performed. The recording can be used during the decompression to assess how the neurolysis is progressing and to help determine if more decompression is needed. Once the surgeon has completed the nerve release, a final recording is made for each muscle using the same stimulus probe location on the nerve and the same current settings (**Fig. 7**). To get a good recording of each muscle, 3 variables need to be considered: location of the stimulating electrode on the nerve, the location of the needle electrode in the muscle being recorded, and the amplitude of the stimulus delivered through the stimulating electrode. It should be stressed that if the surgeon is having difficulty getting a good recording from the muscle at the beginning of the process, the recording needle electrode should be moved. The process for this is to use 1 hand to stimulate the nerve with the stimulating electrode and the other hand to move the position of the recording electrode in the muscle. While doing this, the surgeon may listen and watch for a larger response on the monitor. To move the recording needle electrode, either remove it and place it through the skin at another location along the muscle or redirect at different angle beneath the skin (**Fig. 8**). Other variables to be considered are the electrodes that are used and the type of stimulating probe. In early protocols, the stimulator

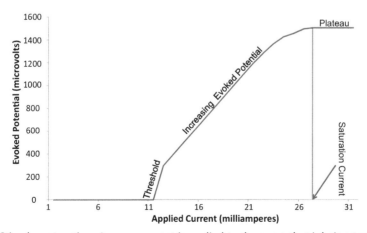

Fig. 5. Stimulus saturation. As more current is applied to the nerve that is being tested, the first evoked response noted in the muscle is labeled threshold and, as more current is applied, evoked potentials increase in amplitude until a point of saturation is reached. This point of saturation is the lowest amount of current that will stimulate all of the nerve fascicles resulting in a plateau.

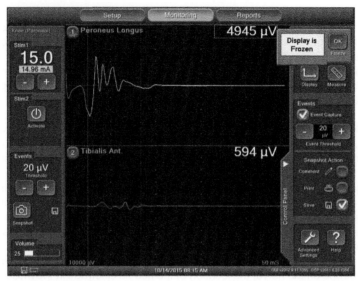

Fig. 6. Common peroneal nerve predecompression. Values showing evoked potential readings of the tibialis anterior and peroneus longus before the nerve decompression.

was a ball-point probe; however, the hockey stick–shaped probe (**Fig. 9**) is more frequently used because it has been shown to more successfully saturate the nerve fascicles (**Fig. 10**). The better saturation is achieved because of the relatively large surface area of the stimulating probe. Spreading the current over a larger area has improved the consistency of recordings. Future improvement of the stimulating probe design and recording electrodes may be considered.

A   **B**

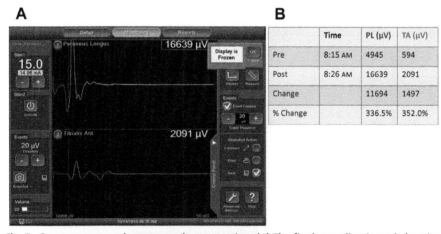

	Time	PL (μV)	TA (μV)
Pre	8:15 AM	4945	594
Post	8:26 AM	16639	2091
Change		11694	1497
% Change		336.5%	352.0%

Fig. 7. Common peroneal nerve postdecompression. (*A*) The final recording is made by stimulating the same location on the nerve at the same current settings. (*B*) Change of microvolts (μV) in the evoked potential of the peroneus longus (PL) and tibialis anterior (TA) between predecompression (Pre) and postdecompression (Post). Note the time at the bottom of the NIM screen shows 08:26 AM, 11 minutes after the predecompression measurements in **Fig. 6**.

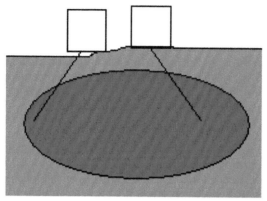

Fig. 8. Placement of recording electrode. To change the depth of the recording electrode in the muscle, angle needle laterally but keep the hub at the skin surface.

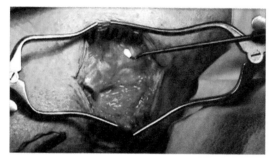

Fig. 9. Intraoperative nerve stimulating probe. The hockey stick probe before nerve stimulation.

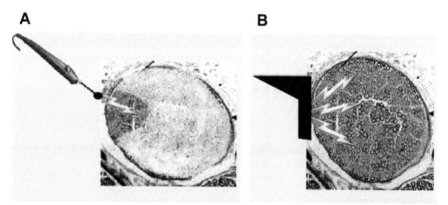

Fig. 10. Saturation. (*A*) Ball tip probe showing saturation of fewer fascicles (*green*). (*B*) The hockey stick–shaped probe increases the surface area and results in complete saturation of fascicles.

DISCUSSION

Once the decompression is completed, it is not uncommon to see significant improvement in the final recordings compared with the initial (baseline) recordings. This is shown in **Figs. 6** and **7** where increases in EMG amplitude of 336.5% and 352% for PL and TA respectively were seen 11 minutes after the predecompression measures were taken (08:15 AM bottom of NIM screen in **Fig. 6**, 08:26 AM in **Fig. 7**). This technique allows the surgeon to gather objective feedback throughout the surgery regarding the success of the decompression. If minimal change has taken place between the predecompression and postdecompression recordings then more neurolysis may need to be considered. In addition to an increased evoked potential after decompression, the surgeon may also observe a louder sound originating from the NIM machine and increased muscle contracture. In cases in which an improvement in evoked potential is not noted after decompression, it is advised to note the improvement of contracture that is visually observed. For example, the authors found that decompression of the common fibular nerve did not yield improvements in evoked potentials for all who had surgery. In a paper submitted for publication on a 40 subject retrospective study, 82% of limbs showed improvement and 73% of the monitored muscles showed improvement. (Dr Anderson JC, submitted for publication.) It is important to note that there were no serious adverse effects (ie, death, myocardial infarcts, or stroke), no unanticipated adverse events, no adverse events requiring intervention, and no adverse events related to the NIM. Although improved EMG was not seen in every case in the study, it is striking that it was seen at all considering it was recorded within 1 minute after decompression and in patients with chronic diabetic neuropathy (mean disease duration: 12.1 ± 9.9 years). Further, recovery of the nerve will continue in most patients and is typically seen in follow-up visits, even in cases in which no improvement was seen intraoperatively. Additional work is needed to develop and implement a rigorous protocol along with improvement of the recording techniques and modifications to the stimulating electrodes. The concept of IONM is still improving and further studies are needed to improve consistency and accuracy.

SUMMARY

IONM can be a useful adjunct protocol to assist the surgeon performing nerve decompression procedures. The surgeon must be flexible in the approach to using it. Initially, IONM can be used to localize the nerve and indicate how successful the surgery was postdecompression. It should be noted that a surgeon interested in using IONM for research purposes needs to follow a more rigorous and strict protocol than described here. Furthermore, lower extremity surgeons will find IONM a useful tool in the surgical arena to provide useful feedback to themselves, their patients, and as objective evidence to document the results of the surgery.

ACKNOWLEDGMENTS

The author would like to thank Megan Fritz, D.C., M.S. and John-Michael Benson, B.S. for their contributions to this article.

SUPPLEMENTARY DATA

Videos related to this article can be found at http://dx.doi.org/10.1016/j.cpm.2015.12.003.

REFERENCES

1. Tavee J, Zhou L. Small fiber neuropathy: a burning problem. Cleve Clin J Med 2009;76(5):297–305.
2. Tesfaye S, Selvarajah D. Advances in the epidemiology, pathogenesis and management of diabetic peripheral neuropathy. Diabetes Metab Res Rev 2012; 28(Suppl 1):8–14.
3. Menke A, Casagrande S, Geiss L, et al. Prevalence of and trends in diabetes among adults in the United States, 1988-2012. JAMA 2015;314(10): 1021–9.
4. Dellon AL. Treatment of symptomatic diabetic neuropathy by surgical decompression of multiple peripheral nerves. Plast Reconstr Surg 1992;89(4):689–97 [discussion: 698–9].
5. Siemionow M, Alghoul M, Molski M, et al. Clinical outcome of peripheral nerve decompression in diabetic and nondiabetic peripheral neuropathy. Ann Plast Surg 2006;57(4):385–90.
6. Wood WA, Wood MA. Decompression of peripheral nerves for diabetic neuropathy in the lower extremity. J Foot Ankle Surg 2003;42(5):268–75.
7. Nickerson DS. Low recurrence rate of diabetic foot ulcer after nerve decompression. J Am Podiatr Med Assoc 2010;100(2):111–5.
8. Nickerson DS, Rader AJ. Low long-term risk of foot ulcer recurrence after nerve decompression in a diabetes neuropathy cohort. J Am Podiatr Med Assoc 2013; 103(5):380–6.
9. Nickerson DS, Rader AJ. Nerve decompression after diabetic foot ulceration may protect against recurrence: a 3-year controlled, prospective analysis. J Am Podiatr Med Assoc 2014;104(1):66–70.
10. Zhong W, Zhang W, Yang M, et al. Impact of diabetes mellitus duration on effect of lower extremity nerve decompression in 1,526 diabetic peripheral neuropathy patients. Acta Neurochir (Wien) 2014;156(7):1329–33.
11. Zhang W, Li S, Zheng X. Evaluation of the clinical efficacy of multiple lower extremity nerve decompression in diabetic peripheral neuropathy. J Neurol Surg A Cent Eur Neurosurg 2013;74(2):96–100.
12. Doikov IY, Konsulov SS, Dimov RS, et al. Stimulation electromyography as a method of intraoperative localization and identification of the facial nerve during parotidectomy: review of 15 consecutive parotid surgeries. Folia Med (Plovdiv) 2001;43(4):23–6.
13. Dralle H, Sekulla C, Lorenz K, et al. Intraoperative monitoring of the recurrent laryngeal nerve in thyroid surgery. World J Surg 2008;32(7):1358–66.
14. Randolph GW, Dralle H, International Intraoperative Monitoring Study Group, et al. Electrophysiologic recurrent laryngeal nerve monitoring during thyroid and parathyroid surgery: international standards guideline statement. Laryngoscope 2011;121(Suppl 1):S1–16.
15. Chiang FY, Lu IC, Chen HC, et al. Intraoperative neuromonitoring for early localization and identification of recurrent laryngeal nerve during thyroid surgery. Kaohsiung J Med Sci 2010;26(12):633–9.
16. Gonzalez AA, Jeyanandarajan D, Hansen C, et al. Intraoperative neurophysiological monitoring during spine surgery: a review. Neurosurg Focus 2009; 27(4):E6.
17. Topsakal C, Al-Mefty O, Bulsara KR, et al. Intraoperative monitoring of lower cranial nerves in skull base surgery: technical report and review of 123 monitored cases. Neurosurg Rev 2008;31(1):45–53.

18. Levine TD, et al. A pilot trial of peripheral nerve decompression for painful diabetic neuropathy. Neurology 2013;80(Meeting Abstracts):P01.125.

19. Kiernan MC, Bostock H. Effects of membrane polarization and ischaemia on the excitability properties of human motor axons. Brain 2000;123(Pt 12): 2542–51.

Rationale, Science, and Economics of Surgical Nerve Decompression for Diabetic Neuropathy Foot Complications

David Scott Nickerson, MD*

KEYWORDS

- Diabetic neuropathy • Diabetes foot complications • DSPN pain
- Diabetes nerve compression • Nerve decompression
- Diabetes neuropathy economics

KEY POINTS

- Diabetic symmetric peripheral neuropathy (DSPN), also distal sensorimotor polyneuropathy, is responsible for a sizable percentage of complaints seen by podiatrists in North America.
- Neuropathy patients may have pain, numbness, deformities, and restriction of motion, which can lead to ulceration, local infection, sepsis, amputation, and death.
- Current treatments are directed at the control of those signs and symptoms rather than minimizing the precipitating neuropathy that is universally present.
- The current paradigm of etiopathogenesis, length-dependent axonopathy (LDA), overlooks evidence suggesting that peripheral nerve compression and entrapment, which is amenable to surgical decompression, is significantly contributory to DSPN.
- Peer-reviewed literature reports subjective and objective benefits after peripheral nerve decompression (ND) surgery. Reduction of pain, increased sensibility, including 2-point discrimination, improved balance, healing of initial diabetic foot ulceration (DFU), reduction in DFU recurrence and subsequent amputation, improved vascularity measured by transcutaneous P_{O_2}, and improvement of nerve conduction velocity and motor evoked potentials electromyography have all been documented.

INTRODUCTION

Addressing podiatric complications of diabetes mellitus is a large and complicated prospect in which important strides have been made; however, it is still a very great challenge to patients, physicians, insurers, and society as a whole. This article examines the magnitude and parameters of the problem and ventures into the topic of

NE Wyoming Wound Clinic, Sheridan Memorial Hospital, Sheridan, WY, USA
* Corresponding author. PO Box 278, Big Horn, WY 82833.
E-mail address: thenix@fiberpipe.net

Clin Podiatr Med Surg 33 (2016) 267–282
http://dx.doi.org/10.1016/j.cpm.2015.12.004
0891-8422/16/$ – see front matter © 2016 Elsevier Inc. All rights reserved.
podiatric.theclinics.com

surgical nerve decompression (ND) in diabetes. Surgical ND is an effective generation-old method, which, regrettably, is still seriously in the academic wilderness. This article reviews the initial clinical insight, laboratory, anatomic and clinical evidence, and germane recent science suggesting the involvement of physical compression in diabetic symmetric peripheral neuropathy (DSPN). This article offers some thoughts on the deep academic skepticism of ND, and the splendid opportunity that ND seems to offer for neuropathic pain relief, avoidance of diabetic foot complications, and reduction of medical expense and societal costs.

The most common nerve problem encountered in foot and ankle practice in the developed world is diabetic neuropathy. Diabetes mellitus is a disease notable for disturbances of glucose metabolism. Neuropathy is frequently present either initially or eventually in the course of this disease, with an incidence estimated at 30% to 70%.[1,2] The most frequent presentation, to which this article is limited, is diabetic sensorimotor polyneuropathy, often termed DSPN, and described as a progressive, symmetric, distal peripheral neuropathy. Stocking-and-glove anesthesia is a standard clinical description.

PATHOGENESIS

DSPN is often explained as a "dying back" of axons. The classic understanding presumes DSPN to be an irreversible condition beginning usually in the feet, appearing later in the upper extremity, and progressing in severity and proximal involvement with time. The theoretic pathologic cause is termed length-dependent axonopathy (LDA), implying that the metabolic disturbances initially and most severely affect the longest axons, and progressively involve shorter axons as disease persists. At the molecular level, how diabetes produces differing physiologic effects based on axon length has not been explained.

DIABETIC SYMMETRIC PERIPHERAL NEUROPATHY COMPLICATIONS

In any case, DSPN clinically leads to leg and foot symptoms, signs, and a cascade of increasingly severe complications, which often lead to progressive debility and life changes resulting in early demise. Early complaints may be tingling, burning, dry skin, lancinating pains, and numbness. Physical changes of calluses, clawed or hammer toes, and nail alteration are frequently accompanied by joint contracture, atrophic skin, local concentrations of increased tissue pressure, intrinsic muscle atrophy, loss of ankle motion, and deep tendon reflex attenuation. With numbness comes increased risk of foot injury and delayed recognition of tissue damage or wounds, allowing progression of deformity or local infection. The infected wound can progress to sepsis, gangrene, minor or major amputations, and even death. The hazards of this dreadful state of affairs have led to efforts at abatement such as the federally sponsored Lower Extremity Amputation Prevention (LEAP) program. LEAP counsels 5 relatively simple activities for diabetes patients, listed in **Box 1**. Primary care providers should attend to initial diabetic foot ulceration (DFU) prevention activities summarized in **Box 2**.

TREATMENTS AND OUTCOMES

Recommended interventions for avoiding the cascade of DSPN complications are based on an understanding that neuropathy is a universal constant; however, its sequelae can be recognized and minimized, or prevented. Repetitive stress on the skin in the presence or absence of deformity and loss of joint mobility can lead to skin inflammation and eventual tissue breakdown generating a wound, with faulty healing resulting in a chronic ulcer. Sensibility loss complicates the situation with late wound recognition and anesthesia allowing tolerance of continued ambulation

---

Box 1
Lower Extremity Amputation Prevention program activities for patients with diabetic symmetric peripheral neuropathy

- Patient education about skin and nail care in diabetes
- Annual professional foot screening for risk of foot complications
- Daily foot self-inspection
- Appropriate footwear selection
- Recognition and reporting of simple foot problems before they progress to complications

---

Box 2
Provider responsibilities for primary prevention of diabetic foot ulceration

- Screening diabetes cases for neuropathy
- Foot examination at every visit and scheduled regular foot nail and callus care
- Referral of diabetes patients for foot self-care education
- Prescription for therapeutic shoes and insoles and emphasis on their habitual use
- Classification of patient risk by Wagner or University of Texas schemes to direct resources to highest risk cases

---

and pressure effects, which prevent healing. The entire complication cascade of neuropathy, ulceration, recurrence, infection, sepsis, amputation, and the treatment options have been reviewed many times, perhaps best by Lavery and colleagues[3] in *Medical Clinics of North America*. Notable facts and figures are cataloged in **Box 3**.[4–14] This is an alarming registry to contemplate.

Box 3
The distressing tabulation of diabetic symmetric peripheral neuropathy and diabetic foot ulceration facts and risks

- 29 million people in the United States are affected by diabetes
- 60% to 70% of these have neuropathy
- 90% of those with DSPN and, usually, their doctor are unaware of it
- DSPN is almost universally present with DFU
- More than 50% of DFU will become infected
- 20% of infected DFU will require an amputation for healing
- Prior ulcer or amputation brings 32% annual risk of DFU recurrence
- A wound precedes 85% of amputations in diabetes
- Worldwide, an amputation in diabetes occurs every 20 seconds
- After a major amputation, the contralateral leg has 50% risk of amputation within 2 years
- Foot and ankle surgery in DSPN carries 10% to 15% risk of wound infection
- In diabetes, a DFU raises 10-year mortality risk 40%
- Five-year mortality after any diabetic amputation is 68%

Data from Refs.[4–14]

DIABETIC FOOT ULCERATION RECURRENCE

Despite best aftercare efforts, the healed DFU most commonly recurs. Provider interventions recommended to avoid recurrence include skin, nail, and callus care, along
with pressure-relieving inserts and shoes. Surgical tendon or heel cord lengthening
and deformity correction are occasionally recommended. Lavery and colleagues[3] estimate that the healed DFU case treated with recommended best care still faces a
discouraging 30% annual risk of ulcer return with 3-year recurrence being 70% and
5-year recurrence being nearly universal. This accompanies an appalling 5-year mortality of 45%.[15] Traditional treatments provide ulcer-free survival with intact limbs for
only 36% to 65% at 12-month review.[16,17] It is no wonder that foot complications are
so greatly feared by the diabetic patient.

DIABETIC SYMMETRIC PERIPHERAL NEUROPATHY AND DIABETIC FOOT ULCERATION ECONOMICS

The economic impact of diabetes and DSPN is massive, recently estimated to represent a $245 billion expense to the United States and its medical system. Around
22.3 million Americans are living with diabetes and at least 6.3 million more are
believed to be diabetic but undiagnosed.[7] Foot care expenses are of underappreci-
ated scale, particularly if a DFU develops. Such costs have been estimated to
comprise a third of all diabetes-related medical expenses.[18] Rice and colleagues[19] estimate that care of foot ulcers raises annual expenses for diabetes by 9 to 13 billion
dollars more than other diabetes costs. A DFU requiring inpatient care can cost
more than $100,000.[20] Outlays in addition to those covered by third-party payers
include patient copay expense, private payments for provider care, neuroactive
pain medication expense, and such indirect costs as lost productivity, disability payments, absenteeism, and unreimbursed family care. It is undeniable that DSPN is
economically a major medical and societal burden.

RELEVANCE AND POTENTIAL OF NERVE DECOMPRESSION

In this dismal scenario of epidemic diabetes, escalating neuropathy and complication prevalence, swelling expenses and social costs, society searches eagerly for
relief. One therapeutic approach to pain, lost sensibility, primary prevention of
neuropathic DFU (nDFU) and protection against recurrence has been almost
ignored by the diabetes and foot care specialists. This is the outpatient surgical
procedure known as external neurolysis, or ND, targeting the neuropathic origin
of the cascade of diabetic foot complications. ND addresses peripheral nerve
entrapment, or compressed nerves, a common secondary physical complication
of DSPN.[21] Nerves enlarge in DSPN due to a sequence of metabolic events,
including oxidative stress and hyperosmolar effects of intraneural sorbitol accumu-
lation.[22] Compression of nerve trunks commonly follows in longstanding diabetes
as enlarged nerve trunks must glide and function in unyielding fibro-osseous
anatomic tunnels, which are themselves stiffened and contracted by advanced
glycation end products in the Maillard reaction.[23] Clinically, these secondary,
DSPN-associated entrapments are present in up to 33% to 50% of this patient
population.[21,24] Multiple peripheral nerve compressions can generate the classic
stocking-and-glove anesthesia patterns described clinically.[25] Given this nerve
and tunnel size mismatch, it is reasonable to consider decompression of entrapped
nerve trunks for minimizing contributions of secondary entrapment neuropathy to
DSPN signs, symptoms, and sequelae.[26] A similar accommodative approach to

nerve trunk enlargement, anatomic tunnel compressions, and entrapment has been applied with success for more than 50 years in the case of Hansen's disease with leprosy neuritis.[27]

DEVELOPMENT OF THE NERVE DECOMPRESSION HYPOTHESIS

The ND scenario in the DSPN setting was first advanced by Johns Hopkins plastic surgeon Lee Dellon. It was occasioned on being challenged by his diabetic patients, pleased with results of carpal tunnel decompression and ulnar nerve surgery at the elbow, to do something for their numb and painful feet. Though NDs in the arm were commonly recommended and recognized as a standard treatment, there was no general appreciation at the time that a similar compressive pathologic condition in diabetes affected lower extremity nerves as well, and might be amenable to similar external neurolysis procedures.

Dellon and colleagues[28] soon demonstrated, with anatomic and laboratory animal studies, the existence of lower extremity fibro-osseous compression sites, nerve enlargement, and entrapment as diabetic metabolic disease developed and progressed in the rat. They correlated these findings with hindfoot withdrawal from pain stimulus and progressive gait and track abnormalities, which could all be prevented or reversed by opening the animal's tarsal tunnel analogue. Based on these studies of secondary nerve entrapments in animal DSPN, in 1988 Dellon[29] editorialized that there was good reason to be optimistic that lower extremity pain and numbness in diabetes with neuropathy could be alleviated by external neurolysis. Siemionow and colleagues[30] confirmed, in rats, greater benefits of ND procedures early in the course of diabetes. The ND hypothesis is represented in **Box 4** and its therapeutic corollaries in **Box 5**.

BASIC SCIENCE SUGGESTS MECHANISM

There are clues to the physiologic processes that may be operant in the diabetic neuron during compression and the recovery post-ND. Dyck and colleagues[31] reported that, although conduction block and diminished vibratory sensibility were induced by compression in diabetic nerve, there was apparent protection against axonal degeneration, suggesting the frequent entrapment neuropathy in diabetes

---

Box 4
The nerve compression in diabetic symmetric peripheral neuropathy hypothesis and consequences

The metabolic disturbances of diabetes can engender peripheral nerve trunk enlargement and shrunken fibro-osseous tunnels, and produce multiple sites of nerve compression and entrapment resulting in:

1. Nerve entrapment syndromes

2. Stocking-and-glove anesthesia

3. Neuropathic pain

4. Diabetic foot ulcers and recurrence

5. Infections, sepsis, and gangrene

6. Life-altering amputations

7. Early mortality

Box 5
Corollaries to the nerve decompression hypothesis

ND in DSPN can

1. Relieve pain

2. Restore protective sensation (1 point and 2 point quantitative sensory testing)

3. Prevent most neuropathic ulceration, reulceration, infection risk, and amputation

4. Improve electrophysiologic function (nerve conduction velocity and electromyography)

---

might be due to pathologic changes not in nerve but in fibro-osseous structures. They report that compression induced lengthening of internodes, obscuration of nodes of Ranvier, and widening of internodal gaps.[32] Jaramillo and colleagues[33] noted resistance of the action potential to inactivation by the neural ischemia observed in diabetic patients. Investigation by Gupta and colleagues[34] (University of California Irvine orthopedic group) confirmed that compression produces demyelination and remyelination in mice, and can be modified by decompression, preferably done early as also shown by Siemionow and colleagues,[30] and Jung and colleagues.[35] Schwann cells can respond directly to mechanical stimuli by proliferating and downregulating myelin-associated proteins like Myo-inositol, whereas desert hedgehog protein limits demyelination.[36,37] Axonal sprouting without Wallerian degeneration is seen at compression sites. Pham and Gupta[38] lead us to think that chronic nerve compression injury is a Schwann cell-mediated disease.

CLINICAL CORRELATES TO BASIC SCIENCE

Dahlin[39] suggested that diabetes may confer on the human peripheral nerve an increased susceptibility to compression injuries. Diabetic nerve enlargement has been demonstrated with ultrasound by many investigators[40–42] and Macaré van Maurik and colleagues[43] showed both nerve enlargement and tarsal tunnel ligament thickening, which supports compression entrapments being contributory in DSPN. Thakkar and colleagues[44] reviewed the MRI abnormalities of diabetes, with early T2 hyperintensity and neural fascicular enlargements, then late atrophy and fat deposition. In diabetic nerves, electrophysiology shows prolonged distal motor latency, slower sensory nerve conduction velocity, with significantly lower sensory nerve action potential and amplitude of compound muscle action potential.[45] With ND, improvements in both sensory and motor nerve function are observed.[46] Recovery room hypersensitivity to touch is common and intraoperative motor evoked potential (MEP) electromyography (EMG) improvements are frequently observed, as **Fig. 1** illustrates.

OPERATIVE NERVE DECOMPRESSION SCIENTIFIC LITERATURE

Dellon[26] reported favorable clinical results of ND in symptomatic diabetic extremity entrapments in 1992. Multiple subsequent reports demonstrated that for DSPN cases with adequate circulation and signs of nerve compression, relief of pain and some recovery of sensibility could be expected in about 80% with proper selection of ND candidates.[47–49] Preoperative criteria should be the DSPN diagnosis, well-controlled glycemia, significant pain uncontrolled by medications, a positive Tinel percussion test, adequate extremity circulation, weight less than 300 lb or 135 kg, and absence of significant pedal edema. The Tinel-Hoffman sign, a distally radiating tingling or buzzing phenomena on nerve percussion at anatomic entrapment sites, is key.[24,48,50] Think

Posterior Tibial n. Decompression
Tarsal Tunnel
Patient 38179 (March 1, 2013)

EMG Recordings:
   Abductor digiti minimi (ADM)
   Abductor hallucis (AH)

   Pre Release 8:54 AM
   ADM: 289 µV
   AH: 125 µV

   Post Release 9:00 AM
   ADM: 1344 µV (465%)
   AH: 781 µV (625%)

Stimulus Parameters (Pre & Post):
Current (1.5x saturation):   9.0 mA
Pulse Width: 100 µsec

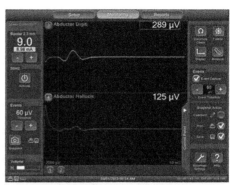

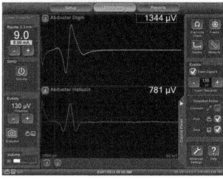

Fig. 1. Greater than 400% intraoperative improvement of MEP for tibial nerve supplied muscles in 6-minute interval during a tarsal tunnel ND procedure. (*Courtesy of* Dr Stephen Barrett, Phoenix, AZ.)

of the sensation produced by smacking your elbow at the so-called crazy bone. Absent this clinical sign, expectation of good results decreases to 50%, still a worthwhile benefit in the responders. At the fibular neck over the peroneal nerve, as well as the tibial nerve in the posterior midcalf, pain or tenderness provoked with digital pressure is counted as Tinel-positive despite lacking radiating tingling.

NERVE DECOMPRESSION SKEPTICISM

The Dellon hypothesis was by no means generally accepted. Thirty years on, it is little recognized and ND is infrequently used. Melenhorst and colleagues[51] report that only 9% of Dutch medical professionals were aware of the possible value of decompression surgery in treating DSPN, whereas 45% reported they specifically explain to patients that DSPN is an irreversible disorder. Only 3% reported they might refer symptomatic patients to a surgeon.

   In explication, many clinicians initially mistakenly supposed that the ND procedure was being touted as curative of DSPN. One might not expect to alter a metabolic disease with a surgical neurolysis procedure. However, in fact, ND was specifically advocated to address only secondary physical nerve compression and to be applied to symptomatic cases only. Neurologists, endocrinologists, and foot-care specialists found it challenging to appreciate the existence of local nerve entrapments as anatomic initiators or contributors to DSPN symptoms, signs, and complications. Many lined up in strong opposition to this thesis as antithetical to the LDA paradigm for elucidating stocking-and-glove sensory change and DSPN.

The published evidence on ND in DSPN was assessed by Chaudhry in a Cochrane Review[52] and a 2006 American Academy of Neurology practice advisory.[53] Baltodano and colleagues[47] point out that these reviews include DSPN cases both with and without entrapment or nerve compression diagnoses. Also, Chaudhry and colleagues specifically view the cases to have either diabetic length-dependent neuropathy or entrapment defined by electrophysiology testing. ND is recommended only for cases with both. Other literature points out the difficulty of distinguishing neuropathy from compression effects in the presence of diabetes.[54] Chaudhry and colleagues concluded that the value of ND surgery of lower limbs for symmetric diabetic peripheral neuropathy is *unproven* due a lack of high-level evidence-based studies such as randomized controlled trials (RCTs). This unproven conclusion has often been misstated by skeptics as *not effective*. Even in the Chaudhry and colleagues[52,53] articles, one can see the misperception of the population and diagnostic target to be treated. It is the secondary, superimposed nerve compression entrapments that are the therapeutic target, rather than the primary DSPN metabolic neuropathy.

Cornblath and colleagues[55] summarized the academic skepticism in the neurology and endocrinology community about use of ND in DSPN. They found issues with of the entrapment or ND approach listed in **Box 6**. Points 1, 3, 4, 5, 6, 7, 8, and 9 are accurate statements but not dispositive of the ND thesis. Point 2 is baldly false. Points 1, 3, 5, 6, 7, and 8 are immaterial to the validity of the entrapment or ND hypothesis. Point 6 highlights clinical observations for which no etiopathogenic hypothesis then existed.[49] Point 7 is purely speculation on future treatment costs. Point 8 is irrelevant. Only points 4 and 9 are pertinent scientific observations that can tested and confirmed or refuted.

Box 6
Critiques of nerve decompression procedure for diabetic symmetric peripheral neuropathy cases by Cornblath and colleagues[55]

1. In DSPN, progressive distal axonal loss occurs, as do sensory and motor signs, and symptoms proximal to the anatomic entrapment sites.

2. Frequency of peripheral nerve entrapments in diabetes is small.

3. The diagnostic Tinel sign, which is not standardized, was initially described to indicate nerve regeneration rather than entrapment, lacks sensitivity, and is nonspecific.

4. Published ND reports are ranked as mostly low-grade evidence from uncontrolled, unblinded, retrospective cohort studies of subjective outcomes.

5. An American Academy of Neurology practice advisory and a Cochrane Review article ranked ND to be of unknown utility for symptomatic DSPN.

6. Immediate pain relief in the operating suite, bilateral pain improvement after unilateral surgery, and 80% to 92% of patients reporting pain relief were too astounding to believe, and no hypothesis for such an unexpected finding was proffered.

7. These treatments are being promoted to patients and could be a large expense to the medical system.

8. Surgical and nonsurgical interventions for other conditions have sometimes failed to fulfill their early promise.

9. Placebo effects, bias, and the natural history of DSPN might explain the hopeful reports of pain relief after ND in the setting of DSPN.

Data from Cornblath DR, Vinik A, Feldman E, et al. Surgical decompression for diabetic sensorimotor polyneuropathy. Diabetes Care 2007;30(2):421–2.

EVIDENCE REBUTS THE SKEPTICS

Overall, recent study protocols are scientifically stronger, with several prospective studies and some level 1 RCTs reported.[43,46,56–61] Evidence has accumulated to provide a valid test of the scientific points of the critique by Cornblath and colleagues.[55] Early clinical ND reports dealt with improvement in the patients' primary complaint, pain, which is a subjective outcome notoriously difficult to measure. Patients' account of numbness, another subjective outcome, was also reported to improve in most after ND.[62] Semiobjective measures of sensibility, such as vibration, temperature perception,[46] 1-point touch pressure and 2-point discrimination,[46] all have shown post-ND recovery, though such measures also depend on patient testimony. Most telling, fully objective measureable outcomes, such as balance and sway,[57] perineural tissue pressure,[63] ulcer and amputation risk,[64] DFU recurrence,[60,62,65,66] hospitalization for foot infection,[62] electrophysiologic improvements in nerve conduction velocity,[46] and EMG values by MEP,[67] all show improvement after neurolysis at anatomic entrapment sites. Especially persuasive is electrophysiological evidence (see **Fig. 1**) demonstrating an immediate 400% improvement in intraoperative MEP of muscles supplied by medial and lateral plantar nerves during tibial ND. This list of 8 positive objective outcomes reported after ND effectively repudiates the point 9 bias and placebo critiques of Cornblath and colleagues.[55]

Baltodano and colleagues[47] reviewed the surgical literature for pain relief, recovery of sensibility, and incidence of post-ND ulcerations or amputations. With the Likert 11-point visual analog pain scale (VAPS), improvements of 1.5 units are considered significant[68,69]; a mean improvement of greater than 4 in 91% of cases is superior to any pharmacologic agents for significant DSPN pain. Their assessment concluded "neurolysis significantly improves outcomes for diabetics with compressed nerves in the lower extremities."[47]

The Rozen DNND (Diabetic Neuropathy Nerve Decompression) Study, just presented and being prepared for publication, ought to provide definitive resolution to the skepticism about using ND for pain in DSPN. This prospective protocol randomized patients both between ND and non-surgical treatments, and also the legs of ND cases to actual neurolysis or sham surgery with only skin incisions. Confirmation of large, durable changes in VAPS for ND was found at highly significant ($P<.0001$) levels at 1 and 4.5 years. And confirmation of large benefit at slightly smaller magnitude was found for the sham surgery, skin incision only legs, a finding pertinent to the Cornblath critique point #6. Macare van Maurick has also demonstrated large benefit to VAPS with ND in a study randomizing ND surgery to one leg and a non-operative control leg in DSPN cases. They too found the non-operated leg also had notable pain inprovements.[59] How this contralateral benefit is produced is uncertain, but its existence now seems ertain.[61]

Such results make the skeptical position increasingly difficult to maintain. In counterbalance to the spectrum of positive results, there are, to the author's knowledge, no negative trials in the literature with a single caveat.

AN UNFORTUNATELY MISLEADING PROTOCOL

Macaré van Maurik and colleagues[59] reported on subjects with painful DSPN who were randomized to unilateral ND in level 1 RCTs. They found subjects with legs that were operated on had significantly better pain relief than contralateral nonoperated control legs. However the abstract of another article reporting balance outcomes of the cohort states, "There is no evidence that surgical decompression of nerves of the lower extremity influences stability within one year after surgery in patients with painful diabetic polyneuropathy."[58] This has been erroneously designated by some as a negative study. The protocol does not actually test the validity of ND for stability improvement. The true finding of the study is that unilateral ND does not improve stability. This is consistent with the Ducic and colleagues[57] initial report finding that bilateral ND is necessary to significantly improve sway and balance but unilateral ND will not suffice. Although this proviso is mentioned briefly in its discussion, the article abstract unfortunately muddies the waters and gives unjustified support to skeptics.

MUSINGS ON PERSISTENT SKEPTICISM

It seems that the skeptical viewpoint continues to depend on the reviews and the Cornblath and colleagues[55] critique, despite its meager scientific footing. The author has heard repeatedly from the conference podium, "There is no evidence," in answer to an audience query about ND and DSPN complications. A diabetes foot care leader recently stated in public symposium that there has been a consensus to embargo discussion and mention of ND as an option for patients for symptomatic DSPN and complications. In view of recent additions to the evidence and literature, this position now seems invalidated. Three decades of delay in settling this question may have done a great disservice to DSPN sufferers in painful distress facing major risk of costly and life altering complications.

The consideration of ND in selected DSPN cases requires a change in paradigm (always a challenging proposition), which frequently encounters strong resistance. A paradigm works until it does not. Only then a change is sought. There is minimal appreciation of the frequency of nerve compression and entrapments in DSPN[21,24] or the benefits when compression is relieved, even though ample published evidence is unchallenged. If a paradigm challenge comes from outside a circle of specialist expertise, its path to acceptance is doubly difficult. Such is surely the case with DSPN nerve compressions and ND, whose proponents must cite from plastic surgery and podiatry literature to persuade neurology and endocrinology authorities. Surely few nonsurgeon experts take the opportunity to observe the indented, compressed nerves of DSPN (**Fig. 2**) recovering normal contour and caliber in the minute or so after operative external neurolysis.

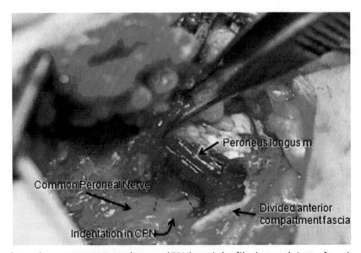

Fig. 2. Indented common peroneal nerve (CPN) at right fibular neck just after decompression by division of peroneus longus fascia and a few muscle fibers. Orientation: patella at clock position 12, foot at 4:30. (*Courtesy of* Dr Stephen Barrett, Phoenix, AZ.)

ECONOMIC VALUE OF NERVE DECOMPRESSION

The potential of ND to have economic benefits in managing diabetes costs rests on reports in of ND protecting against primary and recurrent nDFU (**Table 1**).

Table 1
Occurrence and recurrence of diabetic foot ulceration after nerve decompression in 6 studies of cases with diabetic symmetric peripheral neuropathy, Tinel sign, and adequate circulation

Report	Annual Ulceration Risk (Follow-up)
Aszmann et al,[64] 2004	0% (4.5 y)
Nickerson,[65] 2010	4.6% (2.5 y)
Dellon et al,[62] 2012	3.8%
Zhang et al,[46] 2013	0% (1.5 y)
Nickerson & Rader,[66] 2013	2.3% (5 y)
Nickerson & Rader,[60] 2014	1.6% (3 y)

Standard 1-year recurrence risk is 30%; 3-year risk is 70%.

Risk reductions range from 80% to 100%. Economic benefit is produced by the avoidance of expense for treatment of pain, DFU, infection, hospital care, and amputations (**Fig. 3**).

Two analyses address Cornblath and colleagues[55] point 7, which presumes worrisome economic implications of using ND. We have already referenced the conclusion by Baltodano and colleagues[47] that ND significantly improves outcomes for DSPN with nerve compression. Garrod and colleagues[70] used a decision tree analysis based on the literature to evaluate the utility of surgical ND versus medical management in patients presenting with DSPN and superimposed chronic tibial and peroneal nerve compression. This model demonstrates the potential advantage of decompression surgery for treatment of diabetic neuropathy with superimposed tibial and peroneal nerve compressions. Given their assumptions from the literature, ND is a "cost-effective strategy for society to reduce ulceration ($P<.002$), and reduce amputation ($P<.001$)."[70]

Rankin and colleagues[71] noted the substantial protection against nDFU recurrence that ND provides and applied the greater than 80% reduction in annual recurrence risk to insurer and societal costs that attach to the problem. By minimizing the contribution of recurrences to yearly nDFU incidence of at least 300,000 cases, ND has potential to reduce annual expenditures by nearly 1 billion dollars in year 5. Potential savings include not only third-party insurance payments but also supply costs, private payments to providers, 20% copay for insured cases, cost of neuroactive pain drugs, productivity losses, volunteer or family caregiver services, absenteeism, and disability payments. Additional savings from initial DFU prevention might be realized if ND could be applied to selected high-risk DSPN cases before first neuropathic ulceration[72] and, possibly, to some neuro-ischemic cases.[73] Technologies that may allow selection of such cases exist today.

SUMMARY

ND for the frequent symptomatic nerve compression entrapments found in DSPN has a 2-decade history of effectiveness and safety in dealing with pain and numbness and now 2 confirmatory pain studies using RCT and a sham surgery protocol. More

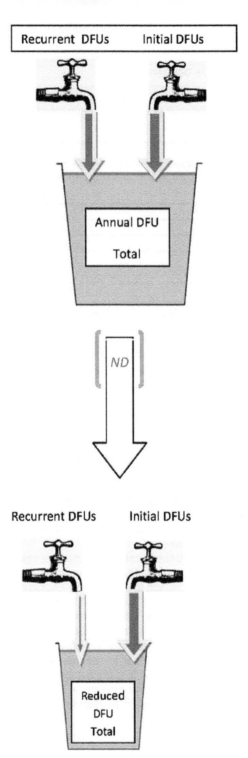

Fig. 3. ND effects on nDFU occurrence and associated costs. (*From* Rankin TM, Miller JD, Gruessner AC, et al. Illustration of cost saving implications of lower extremity nerve decompression to prevent recurrence of diabetic foot ulceration. J Diabetes Sci Technol 2015;9(4):874; with permission.)

recently, evidence of balance and stability improvements and protection against DFU and its complication cascade has accumulated. This proffers significant potential to help contain the large socioeconomic costs of diabetes. Advancing understanding of the results of nerve compression and the basis of altered axonal activity in diabetes clarify how clinical benefit may be occurring. Clinicians should seek to recognize nerve entrapments in their DSPN patients and consider advising ND for relief of symptoms and prevention of complications.

REFERENCES

1. Halawa MR, Karawagh A, Zeidan A, et al. Prevalence of painful diabetic peripheral neuropathy among patients suffering from diabetes mellitus in Saudi Arabia. Curr Med Res Opin 2010;26(2):337–43.
2. Salvotelli L, Stoico V, Perrone F, et al. Prevalence of neuropathy in type 2 diabetic patients and its association with other diabetes complications: The Verona Diabetic Foot Screening Program. J Diabetes Complications 2015;29(8):1066–70.
3. Lavery LA, La Fontaine J, Kim PJ. Preventing the first or recurrent ulcers. Med Clin North Am 2013;97(5):807–20.
4. Lavery LA, Armstrong DG, Wunderlich RP, et al. Risk factors for foot infections in individuals with diabetes. Diabetes Care 2006;29(6):1288–93.
5. Armstrong DG, Lavery LA. Diabetic foot ulcers: prevention, diagnosis and classification. Am Fam Physician 1998;57(6):1325–32, 1337–8.
6. Iversen MM, Tell GS, Riise T, et al. History of foot ulcer increases mortality among individuals with diabetes: ten-year follow-up of the Nord-Trøndelag Health Study, Norway. Diabetes Care 2009;32(12):2193–9.
7. American Diabetes Association. Economic costs of diabetes in the U.S. in 2012. Diabetes Care 2013;36(4):1033–46.
8. Singh N, Armstrong DG, Lipsky BA. Preventing foot ulcers in patients with diabetes. JAMA 2005;293(2):217–28.
9. Morbach S, Furchert H, Groblinghoff U, et al. Long-term prognosis of diabetic foot patients and their limbs: amputation and death over the course of a decade. Diabetes Care 2012;35(10):2021–7.
10. Bongaerts BW, Rathmann W, Heier M, et al. Older subjects with diabetes and prediabetes are frequently unaware of having distal sensorimotor polyneuropathy: the KORA F4 study. Diabetes Care 2013;36(5):1141–6.
11. Wukich DK, Crim BE, Frykberg RG, et al. Neuropathy and poorly controlled diabetes increase the rate of surgical site infection after foot and ankle surgery. J Bone Joint Surg Am 2014;96(10):832–9.
12. Wukich DK, McMillen RL, Lowery NJ, et al. Surgical site infections after foot and ankle surgery: a comparison of patients with and without diabetes. Diabetes Care 2011;34(10):2211–3.
13. Armstrong DG, Lavery LA, Stern S, et al. Is prophylactic diabetic foot surgery dangerous? J Foot Ankle Surg 1996;35(6):585–9.
14. Wukich DK, Lowery NJ, McMillen RL, et al. Postoperative infection rates in foot and ankle surgery: a comparison of patients with and without diabetes mellitus. J Bone Joint Surg Am 2010;92(2):287–95.
15. Martins-Mendes D, Monteiro-Soares M, Boyko EJ, et al. The independent contribution of diabetic foot ulcer on lower extremity amputation and mortality risk. J Diabetes Complications 2014;28(5):632–8.
16. Pound N, Chipchase S, Treece K, et al. Ulcer-free survival following management of foot ulcers in diabetes. Diabet Med 2005;22(10):1306–9.

17. Won SH, Chung CY, Park MS, et al. Risk factors associated with amputation-free survival in patient with diabetic foot ulcers. Yonsei Med J 2014;55(5):1373–8.

18. Driver VR, Fabbi M, Lavery LA, et al. The costs of diabetic foot: the economic case for the limb salvage team. J Am Podiatr Med Assoc 2010;100(5):335–41.

19. Rice JB, Desai U, Cummings AK, et al. Burden of diabetic foot ulcers for Medicare and private insurers. Diabetes Care 2014;37(3):651–8.

20. Skrepnek GH, Armstrong DG, Mills JL. Open bypass and endovascular procedures among diabetic foot ulcer cases in the United States from 2001 to 2010. J Vasc Surg 2014;60(5):1255–64.

21. Vinik A, Mehrabyan A, Colen L, et al. Focal entrapment neuropathies in diabetes. Diabetes Care 2004;27(7):1783–8.

22. Sessions J, Nickerson DS. Biologic basis of nerve decompression surgery for focal entrapments in diabetic peripheral neuropathy. J Diabetes Sci Technol 2014;8(2):412–8.

23. Thorpe SR, Baynes JW. Role of the Maillard reaction in diabetes mellitus and diseases of aging. Drugs Aging 1996;9(2):69–77.

24. Shar Hashemi S, Cheikh I, Lee Dellon A. Prevalence of upper and lower extremity Tinel signs in diabetics: cross-sectional study from a United States, urban hospital-based population. J Diabetes Metab 2013;4(245):2.

25. Dellon AL. Diabetic neuropathy: medical and surgical approaches. Clin Podiatr Med Surg 2007;24(3):425–48, viii.

26. Dellon AL. Treatment of symptomatic diabetic neuropathy by surgical decompression of multiple peripheral nerves. Plast Reconstr Surg 1992;89(4):689–97 [discussion: 698–9].

27. Nickerson DS, Nickerson DE. A review of therapeutic nerve decompression for neuropathy in Hansen's disease with research suggestions. J Reconstr Microsurg 2010;26(4):277–84.

28. Dellon AL, Mackinnon SE, Seiler WA 4th. Susceptibility of the diabetic nerve to chronic compression. Ann Plast Surg 1988;20(2):117–9.

29. Dellon AL. A cause for optimism in diabetic neuropathy. Ann Plast Surg 1988; 20(2):103–5.

30. Siemionow M, Sari A, Demir Y. Effect of early nerve release on the progression of neuropathy in diabetic rats. Ann Plast Surg 2007;59(1):102–8.

31. Dyck PJ, Engelstad JK, Giannini C, et al. Resistance to axonal degeneration after nerve compression in experimental diabetes. Proc Natl Acad Sci U S A 1989; 86(6):2103–6.

32. Dyck PJ, Lais AC, Giannini C, et al. Structural alterations of nerve during cuff compression. Proc Natl Acad Sci U S A 1990;87(24):9828–32.

33. Jaramillo J, Simard-Duquesne N, Dvornik D. Resistance of the diabetic rat nerve to ischemic inactivation. Can J Physiol Pharmacol 1985;63(7):773–7.

34. Gupta R, Rowshan K, Chao T, et al. Chronic nerve compression induces local demyelination and remyelination in a rat model of carpal tunnel syndrome. Exp Neurol 2004;187(2):500–8.

35. Jung J, Hahn P, Choi B, et al. Early surgical decompression restores neurovascular blood flow and ischemic parameters in an in vivo animal model of nerve compression injury. J Bone Joint Surg Am 2014;96(11):897–906.

36. Tapadia M, Mozaffar T, Gupta R. Compressive neuropathies of the upper extremity: update on pathophysiology, classification, and electrodiagnostic findings. J Hand Surg 2010;35(4):668–77.

37. Jung J, Frump D, Su J, et al. Desert hedgehog is a mediator of demyelination in compression neuropathies. Exp Neurol 2015;271:84–94.

38. Pham K, Gupta R. Understanding the mechanisms of entrapment neuropathies. Review article. Neurosurg Focus 2009;26(2):E7.
39. Dahlin LB. Aspects on pathophysiology of nerve entrapments and nerve compression injuries. Neurosurg Clin N Am 1991;2(1):21–9.
40. Lee D, Dauphinee DM. Morphological and functional changes in the diabetic peripheral nerve: using diagnostic ultrasound and neurosensory testing to select candidates for nerve decompression. J Am Podiatr Med Assoc 2005;95(5):433–7.
41. Riazi S, Bril V, Perkins BA, et al. Can ultrasound of the tibial nerve detect diabetic peripheral neuropathy? A cross-sectional study. Diabetes Care 2012;35(12):2575–9.
42. Zhong W, Zhang W, Yang M, et al. Impact of diabetes mellitus duration on effect of lower extremity nerve decompression in 1,526 diabetic peripheral neuropathy patients. Acta Neurochir (Wien) 2014;156(7):1329–33.
43. Macaré van Maurik JF, Schouten ME, ten Katen I, et al. Ultrasound findings after surgical decompression of the tarsal tunnel in patients with painful diabetic polyneuropathy: a prospective randomized study. Diabetes Care 2014;37(3):767–72.
44. Thakkar RS, Del Grande F, Thawait GK, et al. Spectrum of high-resolution MRI findings in diabetic neuropathy. AJR Am J Roentgenology 2012;199(2):407–12.
45. Zhang Y, Li J, Wang T, et al. Amplitude of sensory nerve action potential in early stage diabetic peripheral neuropathy: an analysis of 500 cases. Neural Regen Res 2014;9(14):1389–94.
46. Zhang W, Zhong W, Yang M, et al. Evaluation of the clinical efficacy of multiple lower-extremity nerve decompression in diabetic peripheral neuropathy. Br J Neurosurg 2013;27(6):795–9.
47. Baltodano PA, Basdag B, Bailey CR, et al. The positive effect of neurolysis on diabetic patients with compressed nerves of the lower extremities: a systematic review and meta-analysis. Plast Reconstr Surg Glob Open 2013;1(4):e24.
48. Dellon AL. The Dellon approach to neurolysis in the neuropathy patient with chronic nerve compression. Handchir Mikrochir Plast Chir 2008;40(6):351–60.
49. Valdivia Valdivia JM, Weinand M, Maloney CT Jr, et al. Surgical treatment of superimposed, lower extremity, peripheral nerve entrapments with diabetic and idiopathic neuropathy. Ann Plast Surg 2013;70(6):675–9.
50. Dellon AL, Muse VL, Scott ND, et al. A positive Tinel sign as predictor of pain relief or sensory recovery after decompression of chronic tibial nerve compression in patients with diabetic neuropathy. J Reconstr Microsurg 2012;28(4):235–40.
51. Melenhorst WB, Overgoor ML, Gonera EG, et al. Nerve decompression surgery as treatment for peripheral diabetic neuropathy: literature overview and awareness among medical professionals. Ann Plast Surg 2009;63(2):217–21.
52. Chaudhry V, Russell J, Belzberg A. Decompressive surgery of lower limbs for symmetrical diabetic peripheral neuropathy. Cochrane Database Syst Rev 2008;(3):CD006152.
53. Chaudhry V, Stevens JC, Kincaid J, et al. Practice advisory: utility of surgical decompression for treatment of diabetic neuropathy: report of the therapeutics and technology assessment subcommittee of the American Academy of Neurology. Neurology 2006;66(12):1805–8.
54. Perkins BA, Olaleye D, Bril V. Carpal tunnel syndrome in patients with diabetic polyneuropathy. Diabetes Care 2002;25(3):565–9.
55. Cornblath DR, Vinik A, Feldman E, et al. Surgical decompression for diabetic sensorimotor polyneuropathy. Diabetes Care 2007;30(2):421–2.
56. Aszmann OC, Kress KM, Dellon AL. Results of decompression of peripheral nerves in diabetics: a prospective, blinded study. Plast Reconstr Surg 2000; 106(4):816–22.

57. Ducic I, Taylor NS, Dellon AL. Relationship between peripheral nerve decompression and gain of pedal sensibility and balance in patients with peripheral neuropathy. Ann Plast Surg 2006;56(2):145–50.

58. Macaré van Maurik JF, Ter Horst B, van Hal M, et al. Effect of surgical decompression of nerves in the lower extremity in patients with painful diabetic polyneuropathy on stability: a randomized controlled trial. Clin Rehabil 2015;29(10):994–1001.

59. Macaré van Maurik JF, van Hal M, van Eijk RP, et al. Value of surgical decompression of compressed nerves in the lower extremity in patients with painful diabetic neuropathy: a randomized controlled trial. Plast Reconstr Surg 2014;134(2): 325–32.

60. Nickerson DS, Rader AJ. Nerve decompression after diabetic foot ulceration may protect against recurrence: a 3-year controlled, prospective analysis. J Am Podiatr Med Assoc 2014;104(1):66–70.

61. Rozen S. Level 1 DNND Nerve Study; Reports and Insights. Presented at the Annual Symposium. Association of Extremity Nerve Surgeons. Wimberley, TX; 2015.

62. Dellon AL, Muse VL, Nickerson DS, et al. Prevention of ulceration, amputation, and reduction of hospitalization: outcomes of a prospective multicenter trial of tibial neurolysis in patients with diabetic neuropathy. J Reconstr Microsurg 2012;28(4):241–6.

63. Rosson GD, Larson AR, Williams EH, et al. Tibial nerve decompression in patients with tarsal tunnel syndrome: pressures in the tarsal, medial plantar, and lateral plantar tunnels. Plast Reconstr Surg 2009;124(4):1202–10.

64. Aszmann O, Tassler PL, Dellon AL. Changing the natural history of diabetic neuropathy: incidence of ulcer/amputation in the contralateral limb of patients with a unilateral nerve decompression procedure. Ann Plast Surg 2004;53(6):517–22.

65. Nickerson DS. Low recurrence rate of diabetic foot ulcer after nerve decompression. J Am Podiatr Med Assoc 2010;100(2):111–5.

66. Nickerson DS, Rader AJ. Low long-term risk of foot ulcer recurrence after nerve decompression in a diabetes neuropathy cohort. J Am Podiatr Med Assoc 2013; 103(5):380–6.

67. Barrett S, Levine T, Hank N, et al. A pilot trial of peripheral nerve decompression for painful diabetic neuropathy. 2013; American Academy of Neurology Convention, San Diego, March 16–23, 2013.

68. Todd KH, Funk KG, Funk JP, et al. Clinical significance of reported changes in pain severity. Ann Emerg Med 1996;27(4):485–9.

69. Farrar JT, Portenoy RK, Berlin JA, et al. Defining the clinically important difference in pain outcome measures. Pain 2000;88(3):287–94.

70. Garrod K, Scott LaJoie A, McCabe S, et al. Prevention of ulceration and amputation, by neurolysis of peripheral nerves in diabetics with neuropathy and nerve compression: decision-tree utility analysis. J Diabetes Metab 2014;5(1):5.

71. Rankin TM, Miller JD, Gruessner AC, et al. Illustration of cost saving implications of lower extremity nerve decompression to prevent recurrence of diabetic foot ulceration. J Diabetes Sci Technol 2015;9(4):873–80.

72. Yudovsky D, Nouvong A, Schomacker K, et al. Assessing diabetic foot ulcer development risk with hyperspectral tissue oximetry. J Biomed Opt 2011;16(2): 026009.

73. Trignano E, Fallico N, Chen HC, et al. Evaluation of peripheral microcirculation improvement of foot after tarsal tunnel release in diabetic patients by transcutaneous oximetry. Microsurgery 2015 [Epub ahead of print].

Common Fibular Nerve Compression

Anatomy, Symptoms, Clinical Evaluation, and Surgical Decompression

James C. Anderson, DPM

KEYWORDS

- Common fibular nerve • Common peroneal nerve • Peripheral neuropathy
- Nerve decompression surgery • Dropfoot • Proprioception • Decompression
- Wallerian regeneration

KEY POINTS

- Common fibular nerve decompression may provide significant relief to patients suffering from drop foot. Motor improvement has been shown to be rapid in many cases.
- Common fibular nerve decompression may be the primary procedure of choice in the different treatment options for those suffering from chronic ankle instability.
- Common fibular nerve decompression has been shown to successfully address drop foot that has resulted from intraoperative traction of the sciatic nerve during hip or knee replacement surgeries.
- Common fibular nerve decompression can increase ankle stability by improving proprioceptive ability on the anterior lateral aspect of ankle and dorsal aspect of foot.

BACKGROUND

Nerve decompression for diabetic and nondiabetic neuropathy was introduced to podiatric surgeons in the early 2000s by plastic surgeons who were performing these procedures. These decompressions were typically performed on other areas of the body, in particular the carpal tunnel area. Notably, plastic surgeon Dr Lee Dellon, a prominent clinical researcher who performed nerve decompressions on the upper limb, expanded his research to include tunnels in the lower extremity to improve peripheral neuropathy symptoms among diabetic patients. Dellon introduced and trained podiatric surgeons to perform these decompression procedures. This

J.C. Anderson has no financial disclosures or conflicts of interest.
Anderson Podiatry Center for Nerve Pain, 1355 Riverside Avenue, Fort Collins, CO 80524, USA
E-mail address: JAnderson@ANDERSONPODIATRYCENTER.COM

Clin Podiatr Med Surg 33 (2016) 283–291
http://dx.doi.org/10.1016/j.cpm.2015.12.005   podiatric.theclinics.com
0891-8422/16/$ – see front matter © 2016 Elsevier Inc. All rights reserved.

introduction, however, was received with skepticism because many podiatrists were unaware or slow to embrace the compression component that could be contributing to patients' neuropathy symptoms. In addition, many podiatric surgeons had fairly limited exposure to nerve surgery beyond decompression of the tibial nerve in the tarsal tunnel and excision of interdigital forefoot neuromas. As more podiatrists began to perform the surgery and research began to appear in the podiatric literature proving the efficacy of the procedures,[1] many more podiatric surgeons began to use the technique. Contemporary podiatrists have evolved from exclusive decompression of the tarsal tunnel to include the common fibular nerve tunnel, the superficial fibular nerve tunnel, the deep fibular nerve tunnel, and the soleal sling to treat peripheral nerve entrapment. A careful physical examination and a thorough medical history determine which nerves are being affected and, therefore, which nerve tunnels are involved. This article discusses the anatomy of the nerve and nerve tunnel, the symptoms associated with common fibular nerve compression, and the proper surgical technique to decompress the nerve.

INTRODUCTION

To properly introduce the common fibular nerve, a brief background on the history of nomenclature may be necessary. The term peroneal is often used interchangeably with fibular; however, the adjective peroneal was officially replaced with fibular by the International Federation of Associations of Anatomists and, therefore, fibular is used throughout this article when referencing the aforementioned nerve.

The common fibular nerve is an important nerve to consider when performing a complete neurologic evaluation in the lower extremity.[2] This is because the common fibular nerve can elicit a host of problems if damaged, including tingling, numbness, or prickling sensations. More severe common fibular nerve impairments can also affect motor function causing gait disturbances, including drop foot.[2,3] These problems, although significant, may be commonly overlooked or misdiagnosed by the podiatric physician. The podiatrist may assume the problem is originating from the lower back, resulting in radiculopathy. The physician may also mistakenly assume that after a knee or hip replacement surgery the common fibular nerve is not a relevant component of the differential diagnosis that could be the cause of a postoperative drop foot. A physician may also misattribute ankle instability to frequent ankle sprains or ligament laxity rather than nerve entrapment of the common fibular nerve. The unaware clinician may investigate the possibility of other nerve disorders, such as multiple sclerosis or amyotrophic lateral sclerosis. However, a knowledgeable clinician who understands both the anatomic nerve tunnel and symptoms associated with a damaged common fibular nerve will be able to implement an appropriate diagnostic evaluation.

DESCRIPTION

The common fibular nerve is 1 of 2 primary branches that arise from the sciatic nerve. The common fibular nerve is composed of the spinal nerves from the fourth lumbar nerve through the second sacral nerve. The sciatic nerve divides into the tibial nerve and common fibular nerve immediately proximal to the popliteal fossa. The common fibular nerve then courses distally and laterally entering deep into the lateral leg compartment over the neck of the fibula. It lies beneath a fascial layer before it enters the lateral leg compartment. There are 2 sensory branches found in this area: the lateral sural cutaneous nerve and the recurrent articular nerve. The lateral sural cutaneous nerve forms the sural nerve more distally, whereas the recurrent articular nerve innervates the anterior aspect of the knee. As the common fibular nerve continues more distally, it enters into the lateral leg compartment. At this anatomic location another fascial layer is present. The fascial layer that lies superficial to the nerve but deep to the *peroneus longus* muscle is the posterior crural intermuscular septum. This fascial tissue separates the muscles of the anterior compartment from the posterior compartment. This anatomic location is believed to cause significant compression of the common fibular nerve.[4] After the nerve exits the fibrous tunnel made of the deep fascial layer of the *peroneus longus* muscle, it divides into the deep and superficial fibular nerves. The deep fibular nerve then sends efferent signals via motor branches to innervate the *tibialis anterior, extensor digitorum longus, extensor digitorum brevis, extensor hallucis longus*, and *peroneus tertius*. The superficial fibular nerve courses down the lateral compartment carrying efferent signals to innervate the *peroneus longus* and *peroneus brevis* muscles. Most of these motor nerve branches are in the proximal portion of the leg.

During surgery, it is possible to use intraoperative electromyography (EMG) to monitor nerve function. In the case of the common fibular nerve, electrodes are placed in both the *tibialis anterior* and the *peroneus longus* muscles. A stimulating electrode is then used to artificially innervate the nerve and recordings are gathered as part of the nerve monitoring protocol. (See Anderson JC and Yamasaki DS: Intraoperative Nerve Monitoring During Nerve Decompression Surgery in the Lower Extremity, in this issue.) It has been observed that motor fascicles located in the anterior superior region of the nerve innervate the *tibialis anterior*, whereas motor fascicles innervating the *peroneus longus* lie more posterior and inferior. These observations agree with results published in 1948 by Sunderland and Ray[5] that investigated the intraneural topography of the common fibular nerve. Conflicting information does, however, appear in the literature. For example, a paper was published in 2007 by Kudoh and Sakai,[6] and then another in 2012 by Gustafson and colleagues,[7] suggesting a location $90°$ from what Sunderland and Ray[5] observed. Intraoperative nerve testing also provides evidence that the *peroneus longus* demonstrates more improvement after decompression than the *tibialis anterior*.[8] A proposed theory that may explain this phenomenon is that the change in traction occurs on the posterior or inferior nerve fascicles rather than the anterior or superior fascicles as the leg changes from flexion to full extension. During cadaver dissection, it was observed by the clinicians Dr James Anderson and Dr James Wilton that a motor branch arising from the common fibular nerve frequently courses along the anterior fibular ridge to innervate the *extensor hallucis longus*. These physicians also clinically observed that in early stages of drop foot the *extensor hallucis longus* is affected earlier than other muscles being innervated by the common fibular nerve. It is suggested by these clinicians that this boney edge may have an additive compressive effect on the motor branch, resulting in this muscle being one of the first affected.

SYMPTOMS

Patients affected by common fibular nerve entrapment may exhibit an array of symptoms that manifest through sensory and motor system abnormalities as well as functional impairments.[9] Patients suffering from sensory impairments may have burning, tingling, numbness, and pain in the region innervated by the common fibular nerve.[10] This innervation zone most often extends from the anterolateral aspect of the leg from just below the nerve tunnel to the dorsal aspect of the foot (**Fig. 1**). A common complaint may also be pain at night when blankets touch the anterior part of the leg or dorsum of the foot. Patients may also complain of having to reposition themselves to be more comfortable. During examination, patients suffering from motor

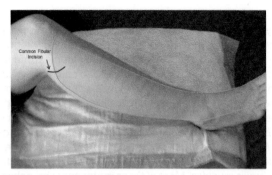

Fig. 1. Common fibular nerve distribution.

impairments will demonstrate abnormalities of the dorsiflexors (ie, *tibialis anterior*) and evertors (ie, *peroneus longus*) of the foot and ankle. Severe damage to the common fibular nerve may limit the ability to dorsiflex and evert the foot (ie, drop foot)[3] and this could lead to a clinical presentation of an abnormal gait (ie, steppage gait pattern). Due to the lack of muscle strength in the *tibialis anterior*, which normally provides an eccentric lengthening function, there may be reduced ability to control plantar flexion of the foot due to loss of antagonistic muscle innervation.[11] This may lead to a very antalgic gait and instability. Patients who do not demonstrate weakness may still present some gait disturbances due to lack of afferent proprioceptive feedback that arises from muscle spindles of the *tibialis anterior* and *peroneus longus*. Lack of proprioception is especially apparent if the nerves being affected innervate the plantar aspect of the foot. This is a more subtle complication than motor weakness and can be assessed using gait analysis and proprioceptive evaluation techniques (ie, Romberg). Proprioception and gait impairment is currently being investigated by the author in collaboration with the Neuromuscular Function Lab at Colorado State University.

CAUSE OF NEURAL ENTRAPMENT

Damage to or entrapment of the common fibular nerve can have multiple causes. They may include trauma to the nerve, including blunt trauma, proximal fibular fracture, surgical complications; or compression from an improperly positioned cast. Drop foot may be a potential complication of total hip or knee replacement arthroplasty[12,13] and the mechanisms of this could be due to the traction that is placed on the sciatic nerve during surgery. Because the common fibular nerve is a distal extension of the sciatic nerve, it is thought that, if damage occurs to the sciatic nerve, the common fibular nerve may be damaged, resulting in a drop foot.[14]

In the case of diabetic neuropathy it has been shown that metabolic nerve tissue is likely to swell as a result of sorbitol in the nerve tissue.[15] This swelling can result in a greater potential for nerve compression in the aforementioned anatomic tunnel caused by increase nerve diameter. In the case of idiopathic neuropathy, the patient may be predisposed with slightly smaller nerve tunnels or there may be mechanical stress to the nerve via bone or muscle.

CLINICAL EXAMINATION

Before nerve testing (eg, nerve conduction, pressure specified sensory device, nerve density testing) is ordered, a thorough clinical examination will indicate if there is an underlying cause for their symptoms other than nerve entrapment. This examination will provide a holistic perspective on how to treat the patient and will also determine if the clinician should proceed with nerve testing. The neurologic examination should assess different sensory modalities including sharp, dull, and vibratory sensation in both limbs. (See Wilton JP: Lower Extremity Focused Neurological Examination, in this issue.) This will determine if there is compromised sensory function throughout the distribution of the suspected nerve. Muscle testing should also be performed bilaterally among all muscle groups to detect weakness or motor impairment in the lower extremities. A gait evaluation, in addition to a Romberg test, will help determine if the patient is exhibiting signs of drop foot or impaired proprioceptive ability, which could indicate common fibular nerve entrapment. A pressure-specific sensory device test could also be used to quantify the patient's sensitivity to pressure and assess their 2-point discrimination. This test may also be performed along with EMG and nerve conduction testing. Lumbar radiculopathy and history of spinal surgery or lumbosacral pathologic condition must also be considered because these complications may present similar symptoms throughout the common fibular nerve innervation area. If the differential diagnosis implies a peripheral neural entrapment, a diagnostic injection may be used to confirm the diagnosis. In most cases, the injection will consist of lidocaine and dexamethasone, and should be injected near the common fibular nerve tunnel. Following the diagnostic injection, a cam walker or ankle brace may be needed to protect the ankle from an inversion injury until the effects of the anesthesia has worn off.

NERVE DECOMPRESSION SURGERY

If the clinical evaluation determined that nerve entrapment is the cause of the patient's symptoms, then nerve decompression surgery may be an appropriate avenue for treatment. Intraoperative nerve monitoring may be used during the surgery and, if so, use of a thigh tourniquet should be avoided due to its propensity to alter nerve monitoring recordings. The patient is placed in a supine position with the knee flexed at approximately 45°. The bend in the knee enhances the surgeon's ability to localize the common fibular nerve and increases the laxity of the nerve to prevent damage to it and promote nerve gliding. It is important to use the head of the fibula as a reference point for incision placement (**Fig. 2**). Palpation of the fibular head may be difficult among obese patients. Therefore, a C-arm may be needed to mark the location on the skin. This extra step will help to prevent a misplaced incision. The incision begins approximately 1 cm distal and anterior to the area where the nerve passes over the fibula and continues proximally from anterior distal to posterior proximal approximately 4 cm (see **Fig. 2**). After the incision is made, dissection is carried down through the subcutaneous adipose tissue to identify the fascial layers over the nerve and the lateral leg compartment. It is necessary to use the head of the fibula as a landmark to guide the surgeon throughout the dissection. It should be noted that there may be more adipose tissue over the fascial layers, which will have a more yellow appearance. The lateral leg compartment will appear either white with a thick fascial layer or as muscle if the fascia is thin. At this point in the surgery there will be 2 defined sections: a more proximal fascial layer composed of 2 layers superficial to the nerve and a defined lateral leg compartment more distally (**Fig. 3**). The fascial layer comprises a thinner superficial layer and a thicker deeper layer that is adjacent to the nerve. The surgeon should be able to locate the nerve by direct palpation or with the nerve stimulator when nerve monitoring is used. The first step in the decompression is the release of the 2 fascial layers over the common fibular nerve. This is accomplished

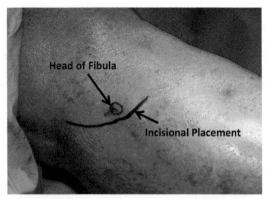

Fig. 2. Common fibular nerve tunnel. Markings for the head of the fibula and the incisional placement for the common fibular nerve.

up to where the nerve passes beneath the lateral leg compartment. The surgeon may also elect to divide the 2 fascial layers using digital palpation and separate the fibers proximally (**Fig. 4**). Once the fascial layer has been released, the second portion of the procedure is performed by decompressing the tissues that form the proximal portion of the lateral leg compartment. As the dissection proceeds more distally, the surgeon must be meticulous to avoid unintentional damage to motor nerve branches in this area. Before decompressing the leg compartment, care should be taken to identify the direction the nerve courses as it dives beneath the muscle compartment over the fibular neck. The dissection should be made directly over the midline of the nerve. With dissection scissors, a release of the lateral leg compartment is then done (**Fig. 5**). The fibers of the *peroneus longus* muscle are then retracted distally and the deep fascial layer over the nerve will then be observed. This fascial layer can vary in length. It should be noted that the tightest region of the nerve tunnel will be here, where the superficial fascial layer and the deep fascial layer merge to form a tight band. This band is the posterior crural intermuscular septum and is the fascial layer between the lateral and posterior leg compartments (**Fig. 6**). Beneath the nerve, there may

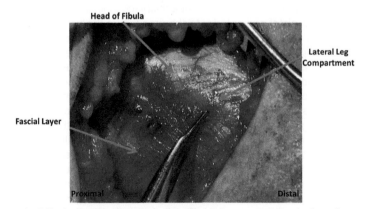

Fig. 3. Head of fibula (landmark). The anatomy of the surgical site before decompression showing the fascial layer and lateral leg compartment.

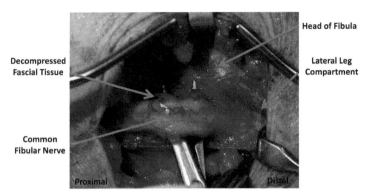

Fig. 4. Postfascial decompression and prelateral leg compartment decompression. The surgical site postdecompression of the fascial layer and predecompression of the lateral leg compartment.

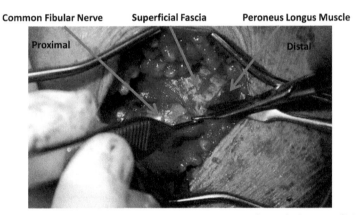

Fig. 5. Decompression of lateral leg compartment. Dissection through the superficial fascial layer over the *peroneus longus* muscle.

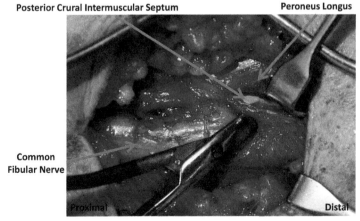

Fig. 6. Decompression of lateral leg compartment. Retraction of the *peroneus longus* muscle distally and the entrapment site of the posterior crural intermuscular septum.

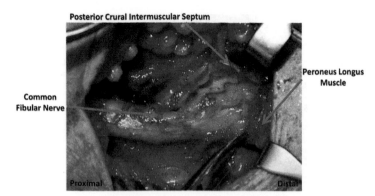

Fig. 7. Postdecompression. Completion of the decompression of the fascial layers proximally and the lateral leg compartment distally.

also be another fibrous band in this same area called the posterior deep fascial arch. Release of this tissue may also be necessary if it is compressing the nerve. At this point, the nerve decompression surgery has been completed (**Fig. 7**). The surgeon should then use subcuticular sutures and a skin closing medium of his or her choice. If a local anesthetic is used, a possibility for postoperative foot drop exists. Therefore, a patient should be weight-bearing in a cam walker to protect them from an inversion sprain until the anesthesia entirely dissipates. Early ambulation is important to reduce potential for scar adhesions that could have a detrimental effect on the outcome of the surgery. These scar adhesions could compromise nerve gliding as it courses throughout the limb, affecting the success of the surgery.

SUMMARY

The common fibular nerve is an important part of the lower extremity nerve anatomy and needs to be considered by clinicians. It is frequently under-recognized. Conducting a thorough medical history and lower extremity neurologic examination is vital. Excellent anatomic knowledge and surgical technique is essential in preventing an adverse event such as a drop foot. Surgical treatment of common fibular nerve impairment can provide for a much more stable and pain-free lower extremity, leading to improved quality of life for the patient.

CASE STUDY

A case study relevant to this article appears in this issue. (See Barrett SL: Case Study – Osseous Pathology with Peripheral Nerve Entrapment and Neuromata.)

ACKNOWLEDGMENTS

The author would like to thank Megan Fritz, DC, MS and John-Michael Benson for their contributions to this article.

REFERENCES

1. Wood WA, Wood MA. Decompression of peripheral nerves for diabetic neuropathy in the lower extremity. J Foot Ankle Surg 2003;42(5):268–75.

2. Sidey JD. Weak ankles. A study of common peroneal entrapment neuropathy. Br Med J 1969;3(5671):623–6.
3. Stewart JD. Foot drop: where, why and what to do? Pract Neurol 2008;8(3): 158–69.
4. Garland H, Moorhouse D. Compressive lesions of the external popliteal (common peroneal) nerve. Br Med J 1952;2(4799):1373–8.
5. Sunderland S, Ray LJ. The intraneural topography of the sciatic nerve and its popliteal divisions in man. Brain 1948;71(Pt. 3):242–73.
6. Kudoh H, Sakai T. Fascicular analysis at perineurial level of the branching pattern of the human common peroneal nerve. Anat Sci Int 2007;82(4):218–26.
7. Gustafson KJ, Grinberg Y, Joseph S, et al. Human distal sciatic nerve fascicular anatomy: implications for ankle control using nerve-cuff electrodes. J Rehabil Res Dev 2012;49(2):309–21.
8. JC A, et al. Acute improvement in intraoperative EMG following common fibular nerve decompression in patients with symptomatic diabetic sensorimotor peripheral neuropathy 1. EMG results. Restor Neurol and Neurosci, in press.
9. Anselmi SJ. Common peroneal nerve compression. J Am Podiatr Med Assoc 2006;96(5):413–7.
10. Boulton AJ, Vinik AI, Arezzo JC, et al. Diabetic neuropathies: a statement by the American Diabetes Association. Diabetes Care 2005;28(4):956–62.
11. Giuffre JL, Bishop AT, Spinner RJ, et al. Partial tibial nerve transfer to the tibialis anterior motor branch to treat peroneal nerve injury after knee trauma. Clin Orthop Relat Res 2012;470(3):779–90.
12. Edwards BN, Tullos HS, Noble PC. Contributory factors and etiology of sciatic nerve palsy in total hip arthroplasty. Clin Orthop Relat Res 1987;(218):136–41.
13. Pal A, Clarke JM, Cameron AE. Case series and literature review: popliteal artery injury following total knee replacement. Int J Surg 2010;8(6):430–5.
14. Baima J, Krivickas L. Evaluation and treatment of peroneal neuropathy. Curr Rev Musculoskelet Med 2008;1(2):147–53.
15. Gabbay KH. Role of sorbitol pathway in neuropathy. Adv Metab Disord 1973; 2(Suppl 2):417–32.

Case Study

Osseous Pathology with Peripheral Nerve Entrapment and Neuromata

Stephen L. Barrett, DPM, MBA*

KEYWORDS

- Case study • Osseous • Peripheral nerve

KEY POINTS

- This case illustrates the complexity and interrelationship of osseous pathology with peripheral nerve entrapment and neuromata.
- The patient had an iatrogenic nerve injury of one of the branches of the medial dorsal cutaneous nerve (superficial peroneal [fibular] nerve) causing her painful scar. This injury likely accounted for her immediate burning pain after surgery.
- The patient developed an injury to her common peroneal nerve from the cast immobilization, resulting in her palsy/drop foot.
- The tarsal tunnel entrapment was likely a sequela of the cast immobilization and chronic swelling.
- The patient's postoperative chronic pain was compounded by the failure to use grommets with the polymeric silicone (Silastic) implant at the initial surgery, leading to a breakdown of the implant with a subsequent detritic synovitis.

INTRODUCTION

Classically, in podiatric surgery, much attention is focused on the osseous pathology; this case illustrates that paradigm. Unfortunately, there can be more than one pain generator present at the same time, which can make surgical treatment decision making difficult and sadly end up with less-than-desirable surgical outcomes because the entirety of pain generation is not addressed. This case is a perfect example of that conundrum.

This case study is connected to the preceding review article, "Common Fibular Nerve Compression: Anatomy, Symptoms, Clinical Evaluation, and Surgical Decompression," by Dr James C. Anderson.

Arizona School of Podiatric Medicine, Midwestern University College of Health Sciences, Glendale, AZ, USA

* Corresponding author. Innovative Neuropathy Treatment Institute, 16601 North 40th Street, Suite 110, Phoenix, AZ 85032.

E-mail address: slbarrettpod@me.com

HISTORY OF PRESENT ILLNESS

DM presented with chronic left foot pain from failed first metatarsophalangeal joint (MPJ) implant arthroplasty surgery 2 years previous to her consultation. She was 39 years old and did not have any comorbidities except for the chronic pain and fatigue associated with her inability to be active. She did have clinical depression and was being treated with fluoxetine, which she described really helped her. She described having immediate burning-type pain when waking up from the surgery, which was still present, and then related that the pain changed in nature about 3 months postoperatively. She was subsequently sent to pain management after her foot became swollen and red at about the 3-month postoperative time frame. She was given a diagnosis of complex regional pain syndrome and began a series of sympathetic blocks. She only had partial relief of her pain and related that the injections seemed to only help for a few days. She was subsequently immobilized with a below-knee cast for 3 months with no improvement. In fact, she started to notice weakness in her left leg and was told that was due to inactivity. She could not tolerate anything to touch her foot and could only ambulate in a walking boot. She was taking more than 100-mg equivalents of morphine daily in different forms.

PHYSICAL EXAMINATION

Because of her allodynia, examination of her foot was difficult. There was swelling noted around the left first MPJ and a slight erythematous nature of her skin. She had difficulty actively dorsiflexing her foot. She could not tolerate even the lightest touch. Examination of the contralateral foot revealed normal pulses, good motor strength, and no hyperalgesia. Proximally, she had a very positive provocative sign of the common peroneal (fibular) nerve at the neck of the fibula. A diagnostic block of the nerve at that location with 2 mL of 2% lidocaine relieved 75% of her pain, which then allowed for her to tolerate light touch. She had normal palpable pulses for the dorsalis pedis and posterior tibial artery. She had a positive Tinel sign of the tibial nerve at the medial ankle and a positive provocation sign, which radiated into her forefoot. Radiographs were taken and can be seen in **Figs. 1** and **2**.

ASSESSMENT

1. Failed polymeric silicone (Silastic) implant left first MPJ
2. Scar neuromata left first MPJ
3. Chronic postsurgical pain
4. Common peroneal (fibular) nerve entrapment left
5. Tarsal tunnel syndrome left
6. Depression

PLAN

Extensive consultation was held with the patient, and she revealed that this was her sixth opinion. The author's recommendation was to replace her implant with a new one, with grommets this time; denervate the painful scar; and perform nerve decompressions of the common peroneal (fibular) nerve, the tibial nerve, and the medial and lateral plantar nerves. She would be managed perioperatively with preoperative gabapentin (1200 mg 2 hours before surgery), a preoperative ketamine bolus of 0.5 mg/kg, followed by intraoperative infusion of 0.2 to 0.3 mg/kg/h and postregional block with 0.5% bupivacaine. She consented to surgery.

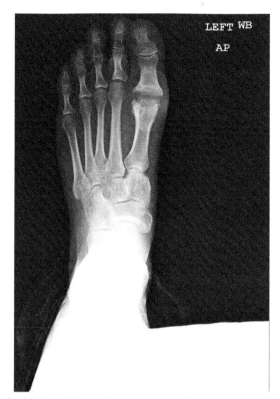

Fig. 1. Radiograph of left weight-bearing anteroposterior.

SURGERY

Procedure: Neurolysis of the common peroneal (fibular) nerve was performed. As can be seen in **Fig. 3**, there was an hourglass impingement of the common peroneal (fibular) nerve. The surgery was performed with loupe magnification of 3.5×.

Procedure: Neurolysis of the tibial, medial, and lateral plantar nerves was performed.

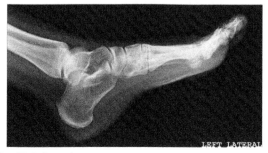

Fig. 2. Radiograph of left lateral.

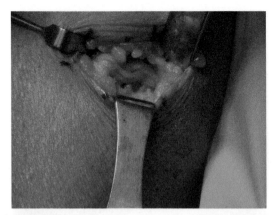

Fig. 3. Hourglass impingement of the common peroneal (fibular) nerve.

Procedure: Denervation of the painful scar was performed (**Fig. 4**).

Procedure: Revision arthroplasty of first MPJ with replacement of Silastic implant was performed (**Fig. 5**).

POSTOPERATIVE

At 1 week after surgery, the patient related surgical pain but stated that she did not have the chronic pain that she had for the previous 2 years and could move her foot again. She was able to decrease her daily pain medications to 60 mg of morphine by day 7. At day 14, she was inquiring if she still had to take pain medications. The author had advised her to gradually decrease them as she had been on opioids for so long. At 1-month postoperatively she was fully ambulatory and fully functional without any pain medication. See **Fig. 6**, which are the 1-year postoperative radiographs.

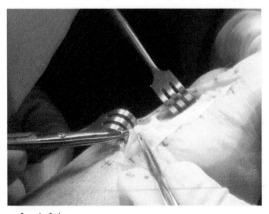

Fig. 4. Denervation of painful scar.

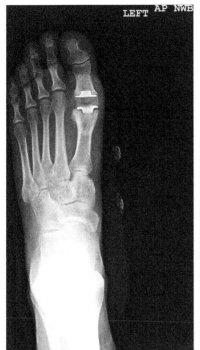

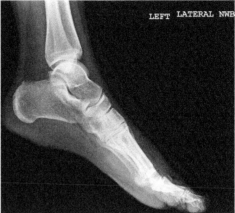

Fig. 5. Revision arthroplasty of first MPJ, with replacement of Silastic implant.

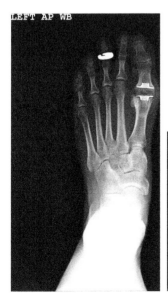

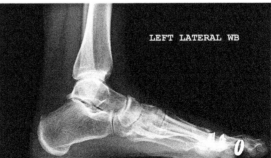

Fig. 6. One-year postoperative radiograph.

Index

Note: Page numbers of article titles are in **boldface**.

Clin Podiatr Med Surg 33 (2016) 299–304
http://dx.doi.org/10.1016/S0891-8422(16)30009-X
0891-8422/16/$ – see front matter © 2016 Elsevier Inc. All rights reserved.

podiatric.theclinics.com

Moving?

Make sure your subscription moves with you!

To notify us of your new address, find your **Clinics Account Number** (located on your mailing label above your name), and contact customer service at:

Email: **journalscustomerservice-usa@elsevier.com**

800-654-2452 (subscribers in the U.S. & Canada)
314-447-8871 (subscribers outside of the U.S. & Canada)

Fax number: **314-447-8029**

Elsevier Health Sciences Division
Subscription Customer Service
3251 Riverport Lane
Maryland Heights, MO 63043

*To ensure uninterrupted delivery of your subscription, please notify us at least 4 weeks in advance of move.

ELSEVIER

Printed and bound by CPI Group (UK) Ltd, Croydon, CR0 4YY

16/10/2024

01775275-0001